A Healthy *You*

ALSO BY CAROL ALT

Eating in the Raw

The Raw 50

Easy Sexy Raw

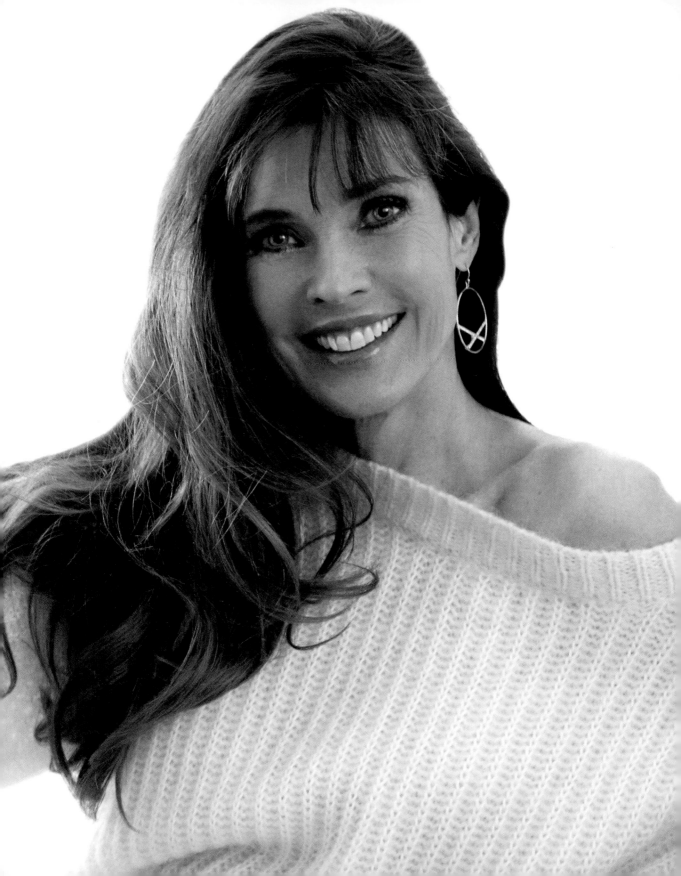

A Healthy *You*

Boost Your Energy, Live Cleaner, and Look and Feel Younger Every Day

---

CAROL ALT

with Jocelyn Steiber

DEY ST.
AN IMPRINT OF WILLIAM MORROW PUBLISHERS

DEY ST.

HarperCollins books may be purchased for educational, business, or sales promotional use. For information, please e-mail the Special Markets Department at SPsales@harpercollins.com.

FIRST EDITION

Designed by Shannon Plunkett

Library of Congress Cataloging-in-Publication Data has been applied for.

ISBN 978-0-06-239297-8

15 16 17 18 19   OV/RRD   10 9 8 7 6 5 4 3 2 1

To all the great doctors who changed my health—and, in doing so, changed my life—and to all the alternative health experts who have come on my show, *A Healthy You & Carol Alt,* to share the incredible information they have painstakingly researched and learned.

Thank you all for your selfless dedication to a healthier way—to trying to find alternatives to pills and surgery.

Thank you for suffering the slings and arrows of nonbelievers to deliver your message and to help other people.

You help me in my quest to pay it forward.

I am forever in your debt.

Contents

Foreword

By David Perlmutter, MD

#1 *New York Times* bestselling author of
*Grain Brain: The Surprising Truth About
Wheat, Carbs, and Sugar—
Your Brain's Silent Killers*

*W*ithout a doubt one of the most important decisions we make on a daily basis is what we choose to eat. And we now find ourselves being strongly influenced, in terms of how and why to make our food decisions, by the vast panorama of recommendations available in the form of books, social media, television, and even advertisements at the point-of-sale.

In broad strokes, these recommendations generally involve varying ratios of the macronutrients (including fat, carbohydrate, and protein), while the notion of consuming foods rich in the micronutrients (vitamins and minerals) seems to be a commonality among most popular diets. Over time, we've seen more and more dietary trends—each one favoring one macronutrient while castigating another. They gain popularity only to be supplanted by the next iteration. Remember, it wasn't too long ago that health care providers actually recommended we reduce our fat consumption under the misguided assumption that dietary fat was somehow detrimental to our health.

But now we understand that simply focusing on macronutrient ratios and micronutrient content represents a significant myopia. The foods we choose to consume are far more than simply metabolic chemicals. Food is information.

Whether our explorations of biology ended in high school or we went on to get PhDs in molecular genetics, each of us was schooled in what has become known as the "central dogma." This basic tenet holds that a flow of information from our DNA directs the production of various proteins that ultimately play fundamental roles in our physiology. Moreover, we were all inculcated with the notion that our DNA was an indelible code that would determine everything from the color of our eyes to the ability of our blood to clot. The statement "It's in my DNA" means the quality in question is a part of a person's essence—something that cannot be altered.

But the expression of our DNA is anything but static. Moment to moment specific genes are being amplified in their expression while others are being silenced—a process that dramatically enhances our ability to adapt to the various environmental changes to which we are exposed. The effect of extrinsic factors in changing genetic expression defines the science of *epigenetics*.

More important, it turns out that these changes in the expression of our DNA, the changes that will favor either health or disease, are to a significant degree under our direct control. The notion that we have control of our genetic expression no doubt seems iconoclastic. But the idea that our choices—the foods we eat, the exercise we get, the levels of stress in our day-to-day lives—influence the expression of our life code should be considered profoundly empowering.

This is not to say that the carbohydrate content or the amount of vitamin C or magnesium contained in a particular food is not relevant in terms of its health implications. But embracing the notion that specific food choices can actually change your genetic destiny will frame your decisions in an all new light. Refined carbohydrates, for example, amplify genetic pathways that increase the body's production of the chemical mediators of inflammation. And now that we've recognized inflammation as a pivotal mechanism in virtually every degenerative condition—from Alzheimer's to coronary artery disease to diabetes and even cancer—the nutritional debate has gained game-changing perspective.

Beyond food, other lifestyle factors also amplify gene expression, culminating in the chemical cascade that enhances inflammation. Stress, sleep deprivation, and even lack of aerobic exercise can conspire to turn on maladaptive gene pathways that ultimately lead to disease.

In the pages that follow, Carol Alt not only reveals her personal epiphany based upon the dramatic lifestyle changes she put into play, but she also draws upon a vast resource of information accumulated during the course of her interviews with some of our most forward-thinking leaders in the area of health and longevity.

My hope is that as you read the text you will recognize that these recommendations can certainly stand on their own when evaluated based upon currently accepted metrics. But from the leading-edge perspective of the epigenetic implications of this program, *A Healthy You* will undoubtedly pave the way for you to rewrite your health destiny.

Introduction

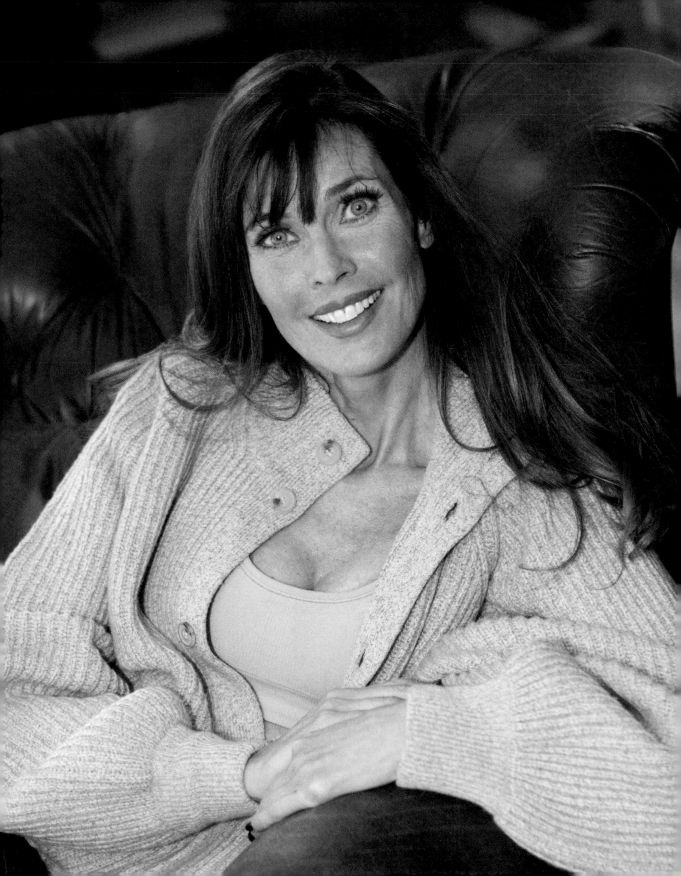

Whether you have seen my television show, *A Healthy You & Carol Alt*, have read my books on raw eating, or have just picked up this book because you are interested in creating a healthier life for you or your family, welcome! I'm so glad to have you here with me on this journey to healthy living. In opening your mind to the new ideas, habits, products, and foods in this book, you've already taken your first step toward creating a healthy you!

You may be surprised to hear this, but at fifty-four years old, I feel more vibrant and alive than ever. I have more energy than I did in my twenties. I jump out of bed each morning not only because I love my career and I'm in the best shape of my life, but also because I am healthier than I've ever been. If you had told me twenty years ago that this is how I would feel in my midfifties, I would have laughed. I wasn't always like this. It was out of necessity that I found my own health and, in turn, my passion in life.

Now I want to share everything I've learned with you!

Discover a Healthy You

Your health is the most important thing in life. It doesn't matter if you have the latest "it" bag, own a huge house, or drive a Mercedes—if you don't have your health, everything else is meaningless. It took me years to figure this out, as I kept thinking I could put my health on the back burner and get to it later. Unfortunately, I realized that that's not how it works! Once I set out to make my health the number one priority in my life, there was no stopping me.

For the past twenty years, I have been an enthusiastic advocate of raw food and alternative health. I'm not a doctor or a scientist, but I

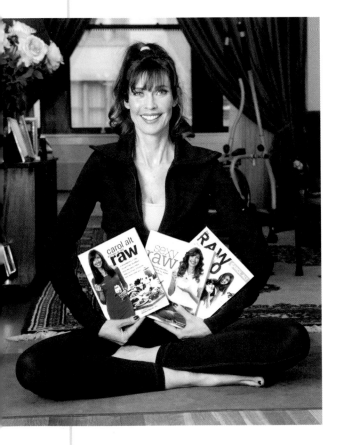

have done a lot of my own research and have been introduced to leading experts in the field—from Dr. Timothy Brantley, who introduced me to raw food, to Dr. Nicholas J. Gonzalez, my current go-to doctor, as well as other amazing stars in the health world, like the *Food Babe* blogger Vani Hari, and One Lucky Duck founder Sarma Melngailis.

I have written three health books— *Eating in the Raw, The Raw 50,* and *Easy Sexy Raw*—to spread the word about the power of raw food, which radically transformed my life. I host my own weekly show on Fox News Channel, *A Healthy You & Carol Alt,* on which I explore natural nutrition, remedies, treatments, beauty, skin

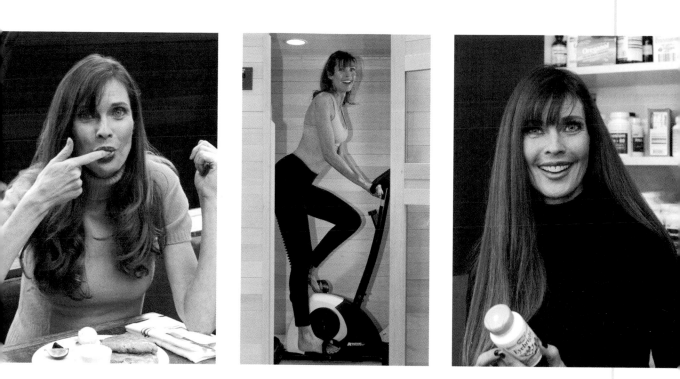

care, and fashion with leading professionals. Through the show and social media I am lucky enough to be able to interact with my audience directly—something that has led me to a greater understanding of the most frequent questions and common ailments that trouble most people. Faced with the same great questions again and again, I realized there are so many conflicting resources out there when it comes to understanding your health. With *A Healthy You* I set out to collect all the best information on common problems and solutions in one place, to help you unlock your true potential.

I would love to tell you that after all these years of research, investigation, working with top doctors, and hosting *A Healthy You & Carol Alt,* I have found the secret to good health—some ancient herb, workout routine or special diet. But the truth is, there is no single product that's going to change your life. You have to take control, create the life you want, and treat your body properly.

Take a second to think about that. While you can't choose your DNA or in some cases your family, town, home, or work environment, you can control your diet, how much sleep you get, your exercise routine, and the beauty and household products you use. I am here to tell you that doing so can make major physical, emotional, and even spiritual differences in your life.

There is no "one size fits all" with health, but my goal with this book is to help you understand your body—to make you feel empowered and in control of your health by introducing you to leading experts who will teach you proper nutrition, exercise and sleep habits, and treatment options. We'll do a little work on the outside too—with expert tips on aging gracefully, makeup, skin care, hair, and fashion, which will help boost your confidence and make a healthier you. I'll also delve into my experiences with these suggestions, some more successful than others—think of me as your human guinea pig!

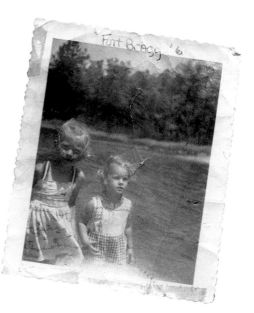

Me and my big sister, Karen.
Notice I was a natural blonde!

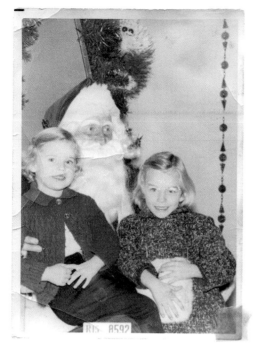

Me and my sister Karen with Santa
Claus, 1963. I'm wearing my favorite
red jacket.

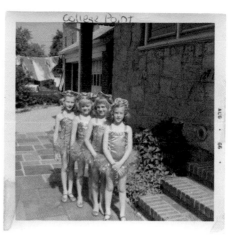

The best thing my mom did for us
tall girls was sign us up for ballet. I
owe all my coordination and half my
modeling career to learning to move
gracefully in dance class. I'm first in
line and my sister Karen is last.

I was the editor of the yearbook in
my senior year of high school. We
took this goof shot of me reading the
dictionary like I was some kind of
brain or something!

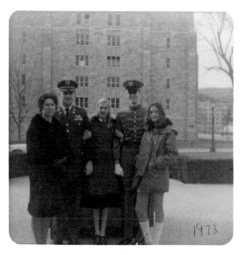

My late brother, Tony Alt, went to
West Point, and going to visit on
weekends was so exciting. *Left
to right:* Mom, Colonel Alt (Dad),
Karen, Tony, and me, 1973.

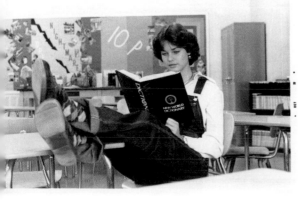

My Story

Like many of you, I didn't grow up with the information on healthy living that is available today. There was no *A Healthy You & Carol Alt* on TV or websites like MindBodyGreen or Natural News that disseminated health-focused information or alternative options. I grew up in a close, humble family in College Point, Queens, New York. Because my parents, as lovely as they were, didn't themselves know the importance of nutritious food and an active lifestyle, they certainly couldn't impart this essential wisdom to their children. I ate what everyone else ate—cereal, bread, milk, eggs, meat, pasta, lots of sugar—pretty much the aptly named S.A.D. (standard American diet). My staples were muffins, baked goods, hamburgers, Chinese food, spaghetti, and pizza. Like a lot of young people, I ate what was convenient. My first few jobs also centered on food. I worked in a bakery starting at age thirteen, and for four years began my days with a delicious hot cinnamon bun right out of the oven! At seventeen, I started working part-time as a waitress and was able to feast on fries and burgers to my heart's content. It was at this restaurant that I was approached by a photographer about modeling.

Me? A model? I couldn't believe it. I knew I was tall, but I also knew I wasn't thin. I was a tomboy growing up, not the type to sit and devour fashion magazines. At the time I was approached, I was attending Hofstra University and had my sights set on a military career. But when I realized that I could earn the same amount in a day of modeling as I could in a month of waitressing, I decided to give it a try as a summer job.

I was immediately told I needed to lose at least fifteen pounds. My solution? I didn't eat much for a few weeks and voilà—I lost the weight and didn't suffer many side effects besides the occasional rumbling tummy. At twenty I felt like I could control my body without consequences, and I was in a world where thin was in. If I was going to be a successful model, I needed to be thin, whatever the cost. Shortly

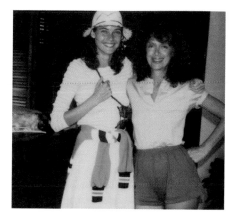

Me and Jule Campbell, the editor of the *Sports Illustrated* Swimsuit Edition, in Port Antonio, Jamaica, November 1982.

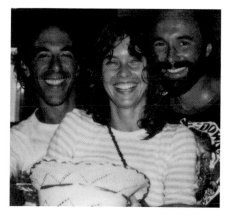

Here I am with photographer Walter Iooss *(right)* and Walter's assistant, Lou *(left)*, on the same *Sports Illustrated* shoot.

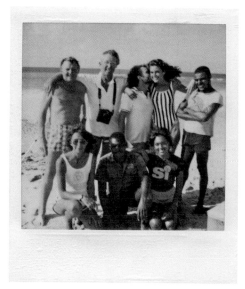

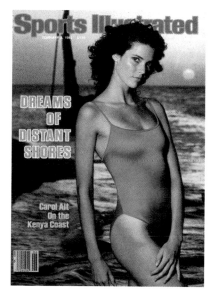

This snapshot was taken in Lamu, Kenya, November 1981. This was the whole crew back then!

Kim Alexis was supposed to be the 1982 *SI* cover girl, but at the very last minute my photo was chosen to replace hers. This was the last shot of the last day of a long trip to Kenya. The boat had just appeared. The sun was just setting. I didn't even have time to comb my hair. And I thought—well, they will never use this shot anyway . . .

after I dropped the initial weight, my modeling career took off. I was flown around the world to shoot for all the major fashion magazines and designers, and of course for the *Sports Illustrated* Swimsuit Edition. To this day, that cover shot still earns me the most recognition.

Still, it was ingrained in my brain that I was fat, so I ate like a person trying to lose weight. For weeks at a time, I would hardly eat anything for fear of gaining weight. My body became accustomed to operating on a small amount of food. Often, I was working such long days that I didn't even realize I was not eating. I would be on a set and by the time I was done, all the food was gone. The crew assumed models didn't eat and put away all the food, so I didn't eat. By that point in my career I had starved myself for so long that I would gain weight if I slipped the slightest bit toward eating a "normal" diet. For years I thought my body was invincible and could handle everything I threw at it—early-morning shoots, skipping meals, rewarding myself with brownies, coffee, coffee, and more coffee, no exercise, and never getting enough sleep.

I learned the hard way that this lifestyle was unsustainable—especially when I hit my late twenties. My health issues started to pile up, becoming unbearable. I was taking cold medicine to fall asleep, coffee to wake up, sinus medicine for my breathing problems, aspirin for my headaches,

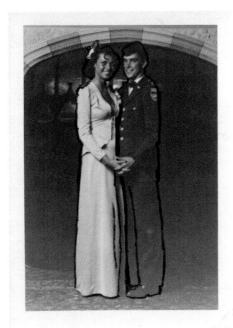

So here is your life, Carol Alt. This was my boyfriend, Michael. He was graduating from prep school in Monmouth, New Jersey, in 1978. I used to take a marker and outline a thinner me in photos to see how I would look if I could lose the extra weight I was carrying.

eight antacids at a time for my stomach pains, and antihistamines for my allergies. I had horrible sugar cravings, a bloated belly, restlessness, foggy thoughts, and sleep issues, and I was very irritable and sluggish all day. My skin became like plastic, and my nails and hair were brittle. I started to dread waking up. I remember hitting the snooze button on my alarm clock at least four times every morning, and the first thing I would grab when I finally did get up was a Scotch coffee with whipped cream (my "secret weapon"—I needed the caffeine and the sugar to get me going). Never once did it occur to me to equate how I felt with what I was eating (or not eating).

I had finally made it in my career, but I felt awful inside. I was hitting rock bottom and I knew something needed to change. I remember the aha moment clearly—I was on the set of a shoot in the Amazon where I was supposed to be the headliner for a "Carol Alt and Friends" photo shoot, and I was exhausted. My morning Scotch coffee did not do the trick. They had invited a twenty-two-year-old model for the shoot and I was amazed at how she shined. I had lost my spark. I looked drained and was hiding behind rocks to cover my belly while this girl was jumping around in a string bikini. What happened? It was supposed to be my shoot, but she was the center of attention. How did I go from a vibrant twenty-two-year-old to a bloated, cranky thirty-four-year-old?

I realized I couldn't keep living this way, but I didn't know what to do next, so I decided to disappear for a while into the Palm Springs desert. The whole time I was there I tried to figure out what was wrong with me. I felt like a blob. How did I lose my "it" factor?

In a twist of fate—and I believe everything happens for a reason—my friend Steven Cantor called while I was in Palm Springs to say hello and check in on me. He had been concerned about my health the last time we had seen each other. As we chatted he explained that his girlfriend at the time had cervical cancer and was fighting it through an alkalizing diet and raw food. He encouraged me to speak with the doctor who was helping her, Dr. Timothy Brantley.

After my call with Steven, I immediately picked up the phone and called Dr. Brantley. He didn't ask how I was feeling, or what was wrong with me—his first question was "What do you eat?" On hearing my reply, he told me, "If you eat like that, I bet you have this, this, and that problem . . ." He went on to reel off my top six ailments with alarming precision: stomach acid, occasional headaches, candida, sinus infections, moodiness, and sluggishness. In fact, he was also able to diagnose problems over the phone that a Park Avenue doctor had misdiagnosed in person!

Calling Dr. Brantley was the best move I've ever made. He suggested I immediately switch to a raw food diet and encouraged me to learn about my body and the food I was eating. This was the first time I had ever been educated on what food can do for your health. Raw food? It sounded a little extreme for someone like me. What about my beloved pasta or chicken? Could I do it? I was at a breaking point, though, and my body was telling me that I needed to change. Now. I decided to "go raw" cold turkey, and after experiencing the life-altering benefits within the first week, I haven't looked back since. Becoming a raw foodist not only saved my life, but it has also led me to discover my true passion—helping other people better understand their bodies and minds and improve their own health and quality of life.

For the first time in years I was eating sufficient amounts of food and, more importantly, the right kinds.

It took a few months to nourish my body back fully, but over time I began to feel vibrant again, and this reflected in every area of my life—physical, mental, professional, and emotional. I no longer had sinus infections or trouble falling asleep or waking up. My headaches were gone, along with my addiction to antacid pills. In short, my body started to heal itself and function like a well-oiled machine. From close friends to new acquaintances, people around me took notice and commented on how radiant and healthy I looked. I may have been a top model, but I had never heard these sorts of compliments before. And it felt great.

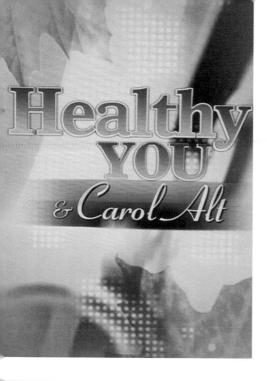

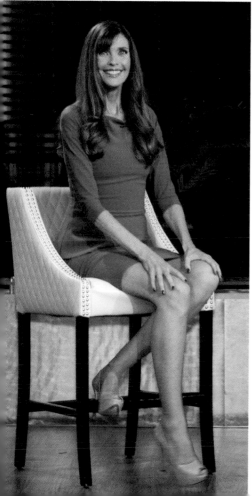

I have been raw for eighteen years and am a living example of the wonders of a raw food diet. I now work with a brilliant doctor in New York City, Dr. Nicholas Gonzalez, who continues to guide and teach me about health. (You'll hear more about him in the Nutrition part of the book, in "Which Diet Is the Best for Me?" on page 32.) Thanks to Dr. Brantley, Dr. Gonzalez, and many other experts along the way, my guiding principle has become that every meal I eat is an opportunity to take a step toward better health.

Learning about raw food has opened my eyes to the wealth of health-related information, and misinformation, that exists. When I started to research, meet with doctors and professionals, and talk to leaders in the health field, I began to see that there wasn't only one option, one treatment plan, when it came to health. There are so many different choices and changes that you can make to impact your life, both today and in the long term. It's about finding the right mix that works for you as an individual. By sharing some of what I've learned along the way, I hope to provide you with the knowledge, as well as the motivation, to make a change, to step forward and become an active participant in your own health. *A Healthy You* offers you the tools for a vibrant life, but it's up to you to go out there and put them into action. Let's do this together!

A Healthy *You*

PART 1
Nutrition

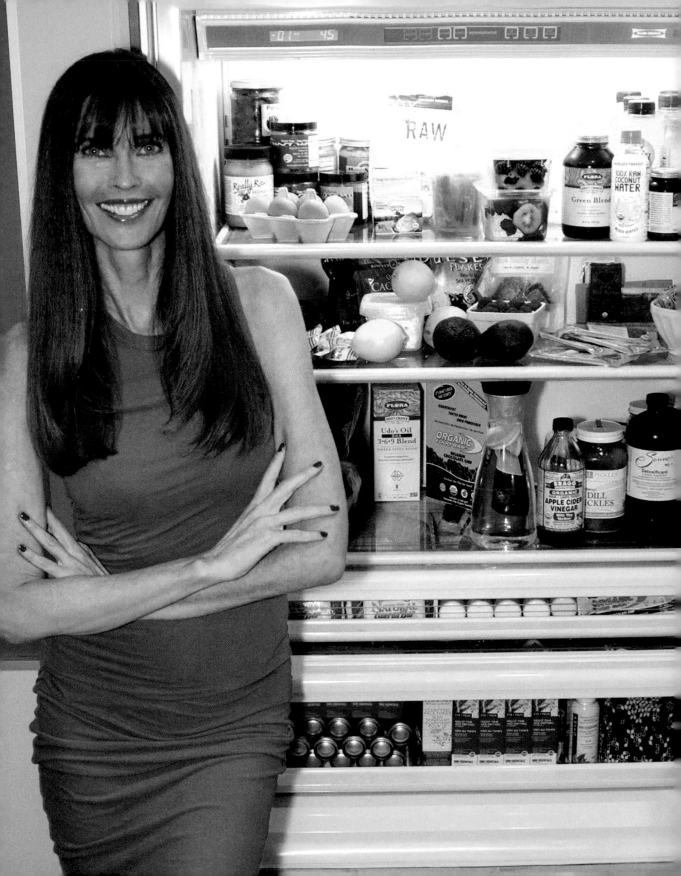

My life changed when I started eating raw and unprocessed foods. I went from being a tired and sick model who was taking medicine for everything, to a vibrant self-confident woman who ate more than she had in years. Through a raw diet, which I'll explain in depth a bit later, I became more conscious of what I was putting in my body every day, at every meal, even when I was snacking. Going raw and eating real food helped me realize that food is the fuel my body needs to function at its optimal level—not something to help me cope with my emotions or to simply make me feel full. When I took time to learn about the food I was consuming and the role that diet played in my overall health, I realized its power. Food, more than anything else, has the ability to heal and mend our bodies. For the first time in my life, I was able to form a different relationship with food—one that focused on the positive aspects of eating foods that gave me energy, boosted my mood, soothed my ailments, and helped me feel alive. What you eat impacts every part of your life. If you change your food, you change your life. Period. It's that easy. I'm a walking example of it!

As you may have guessed, I'm a huge advocate of eating raw food, but I realize this isn't for everyone. I'm going to make the case for raw—I always do!—but you will also learn about the life-changing power of eating real, unprocessed food. Simply cutting out processed foods may be a somewhat less daunting starting point for those of you who are looking to eat a cleaner, healthier diet. In this part of the book, I will explore our all-important relationship with food, and also investigate trends in diet and nutrition that I've come to learn about through interviews I've done with some of my favorite leading doctors and experts. They have all helped to open my eyes to new possibilities on the journey to healthy eating—and I can't wait to share what I've learned with you.

Get ready for tips on which diet is best for you, along with information on cancer-fighting and cancer-preventing foods, alkaline water, my thoughts on the infamous coffee debate, how to grocery shop for success, juicing and blending, and so much more!

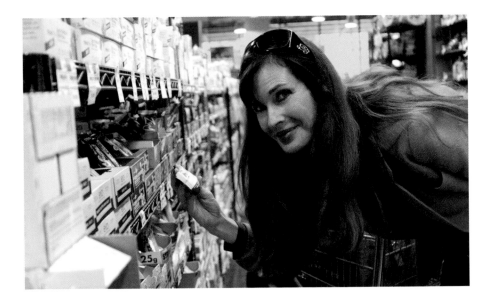

Why Food Matters:
You Are What You Eat

When I was modeling, food was either my best friend or my worst enemy. I would not eat all day for fear of gaining weight, and then, if something went well, I would reward myself with brownies. I needed the sugar to keep me going. I was eating based on my emotions and always feeling guilty. Going raw and educating myself about food helped me change this mind-set. I learned that food is fuel and what we choose affects everything: our bodies, minds, moods, job performance, and relationships—even our sex lives. As they say in Silicon Valley: garbage in, garbage out. In order to fuel myself properly I needed to eat food in its real and natural state. That meant no more garbage in—no more artificial ingredients or processed foods.

You really are what you eat. We've all heard this phrase before, but it doesn't always resonate. Why not? It's so simple. Instead, people are constantly scanning diet and self-help books for the secret formula or product that is going to change their lives. Fad diets and of-the-moment superfoods become popular overnight. We all want a quick fix. We want a smoothie that will knock off five pounds or a green vegetable we can sneak into our otherwise poor diets that will magically make us healthy. The problem is, it doesn't work like that. There is no miracle food or single diet that will take care of all your woes overnight; there is no such thing as a quick fix for your health.

If you eat fast food, chips, candy, or any processed food, your body is going to let you know that it is unhappy! Although they might taste delicious, these types of food do not have any nutritional value, so your body has to go into digestive overdrive to process and metabolize them. Your pancreas will churn out large doses of insulin to break down and absorb all the sugar or processed fat, causing spikes in your blood sugar that can leave you feeling tired, cranky, bloated, and sluggish. The nutrients in your food determine the way your body functions and how your cells develop and thrive. Without proper nutrients, cells become weak and ultimately diseased. You are the accumulation of everything you do to your body—nothing happens all of a sudden, especially when it comes to diet.

Keep in mind that the food you eat every day is an area where you have complete power. You can't control everything in life, but with some planning and thought you can control what you eat. Don't get me wrong, better health through nutrition will take some work: learning about different foods, pushing yourself to try new things, keeping an open mind, and food planning and preparation are all keys for success. But remember, feeding yourself quality, unprocessed food is an investment in your own happiness—choose to feed your body properly, with real food, and it will function at its best! Every meal is an opportunity to take a step toward better health.

Carol's Tip

Try to keep gum chewing to a minimum. Chewing gum signals the digestive system to start breaking down food. Continually starting and stopping your system can be stressful on the body, plus your body wastes enzymes that are not actually needed for digestion.

Raw Made Simple

"OKAY, CAROL, WHAT IS RAW FOOD?"

I'm glad you asked! Raw food is my favorite topic of discussion. If you have read any of my books or watched my show, you are probably familiar with my love for raw food. I just can't keep it to myself, since raw food has done wonders for my life! But if you've never heard the term before, let me explain.

Simply put, raw food is in its natural, unprocessed, and uncooked state. A raw food diet is one that consists of uncooked or dehydrated vegetables, fruits, nuts, seeds, sprouts, fresh herbs, spices, fermented foods, and seaweed. I even eat raw fish and meat.

The key is that no food should be heated above 115°F. Why 115°F? In order for your body to function properly and grow, repair, and maintain itself, it needs enzymes, vitamins, minerals, phytonutrients, essential fats, and fiber. These are all provided by the food you eat. When foods are baked or cooked (heated), many of these key components are altered or destroyed. Without them, your body requires more energy and bodily resources to properly process and digest the food you eat.

Another problem with cooking food is that heating it breaks the unique bond between vitamins and minerals, which is heat-sensitive and deteriorates at high temperatures. Vitamins help regulate your metabolism, convert fat and carbohydrates into energy, and assist in forming bone and tissue. Minerals have a symbiotic relationship with vitamins: they help each other out. Without vitamins and minerals our cells do not function properly and our organs will eventually fail. The body absorbs vitamins and minerals much more readily and easily if they are attached to each other. For example, it's well known that we absorb calcium better when it's grouped with vitamin D and magnesium. That's why most supplements with calcium have vitamin D and magnesium added—to help with absorption. The same thing happens with every vitamin and mineral in our food. Raw food has these vitamins and minerals intact. Vitamins and minerals are simply more bioavailable in raw food. And that's a good thing—a very good thing!

For example, vitamin E protects your cell membranes from damage caused by free radicals (this means your skin cells as well), is an antioxidant, and helps in enzymatic activities. Copper plays a key role in the maintenance of healthy skin and hair. Copper helps produce the skin pigment melanin, which colors the skin, hair, and eyes. When hair turns gray, it may be due to copper deficiency. Would you knowingly want to deprive your body of the exact things that are keeping you looking young and vibrant? And this is only one vitamin and one mineral!

Additionally, when you heat food, you destroy the enzymes that are naturally present in it. Enzymes are the key to life; they drive every chemical reaction in your body. Whenever you eat, salivary glands and certain specialized cells in the stomach, small intestine, and pancreas secrete enzymes, which immediately go to work breaking down the food in your stomach.

However, their job doesn't end there. Enzymes are the living proteins that direct life force into our biochemical and metabolic processes. They help transform and store energy, make active hormones, dissolve fiber, and prevent clotting. They also have anti-inflammatory effects and help balance and restore your immune system, among a myriad of other jobs. A diet rich in enzymes can increase energy and stamina, as well as support healthy skin, weight loss, and overall good health.

You can see how vitally important these vitamins, minerals, and enzymes are in helping to keep your body regenerating and rejuvenated. Why would you want to take the chance of them being less

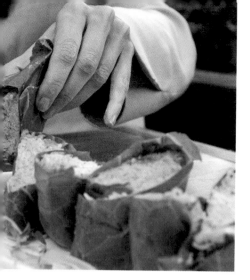

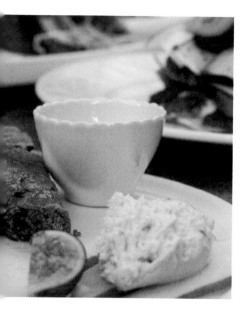

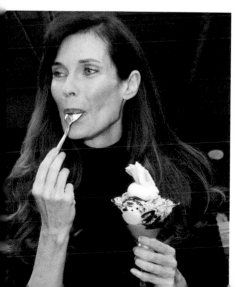

available to your body by denaturing them with heat?

But I didn't stop there. I asked Christopher Dobrowolski, the founder of Live Live & Organic, a raw food market and resource center based in New York City, to talk about some of the chemicals that are present in heated foods but not in raw. He explained that high levels of polyaromatic hydrocarbons (PAHs), by-products of fuel burning, are found in many cooked foods—for example, meat cooked at high temperatures and smoked fish. PAHs are cause for concern because some of them have been identified as carcinogenic. Also, much of the cooked food we eat contains acrylamide, a naturally occurring chemical compound found in many plant-based, high-carbohydrate foods after they've been heated at a high temperature. This chemical, which is also used in the treatment of sewage and waste to manufacture certain chemicals, plastics, and dyes, has been known to cause gene mutations that lead to a range of cancers in rats. Yuck!

"BUT EATING RAW IS TOO HARD!"

This is the first comment I get every time I encourage people to add more raw food to their diets. Being raw doesn't mean giving up everything, nor does it mean going vegan or even vegetarian; you can still eat raw milk cheeses, raw fish or ceviche, and even raw meat in the form of tartare, carpaccio, bresaola, or prosciutto. As nutrition expert David Wolfe has always told me: raw food is about abundance.

When I first started eating raw in the early 1990s, there were no Raw Revolution bars at the local grocery store, or restaurants like

These fabulous desserts are from Pure Food and Wine. And yes, the chocolate is raw and very healthy for you—bioflavonoids and antioxidants abound in raw chocolate.

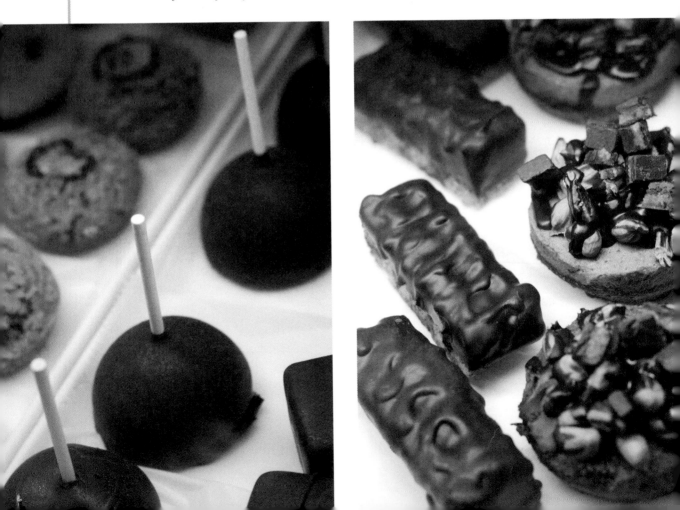

Pure Food and Wine in New York City or any of the countless other restaurants around the globe that now serve only raw food.

Carol's Tip

Check out www.happycow.net for a list of raw or healthy restaurants all around the world.

I had to learn how to prepare food on my own and how to choose wisely when I went out to eat. One of the best consequences of the lack of healthy convenience foods was that I developed an actual relationship with the food I was eating. I started to become more aware of exactly what I was putting in my body as fuel. A red grapefruit wasn't just a piece of fruit—it was a carrier of vitamin C to support my immune system and a source of lycopene, which helps fight cancer. My raw kale salad was filled with fiber, flavonoids, proteins, and vitamins—like beta-carotene and vitamins C, K, and B_6—which would help my body to detox as well as boost my skin, vision, and metabolism, and help me avoid chronic inflammation. And that is just kale! I began to think of food as the source of energy that my body needed instead of a tasty reward for getting through the day. Through a raw diet, I realized I could eat breakfast, lunch, dinner, and a snack without gaining weight. I was eating more food than I had in years. I felt more energized and free than ever before.

Now going raw is easier than many people think. And trust me, the impact it will have on your everyday life will make any of the extra planning and prepping totally worth it. You probably already eat a lot of raw food but don't even realize it. Do you eat salad and fruit? Well, these are raw! It's the label "raw" that scares people. It doesn't have to be scary, though. Start small with one raw meal or snack a day. It's easy to purchase raw snacks online or at your local health-food store. We are lucky to live in a time where these types of stores are more readily available. If you find you like the food, take the next step and try a recipe—in this book I've included a few easy recipes and a breakfast, lunch, dinner, and dessert from my favorite raw foodies.

Carol's Tip

Watch out, not all cold foods are raw. If the label doesn't use a word such as "unprocessed," "raw," "unrefined," or "cold processed," the food might not be raw. Examples of foods that people think are raw but are not include some pickles, olives, hummus, cheeses, milk, butter, yogurt . . . well, you get the drift. No raw label—don't buy it!

Another big question is "How can you be raw and go out to dinner? What happens to your social life?" It's quite easy. A little planning goes a long way. When I go to a restaurant I often check out the menu online before I leave the house to see if they have meals that I like to eat—restaurants always have salads. Don't be shy to ask for the kitchen to remove the chicken or croutons. These days, many menus also carry raw alternatives permanently on the menu, including ceviche, tartare, carpaccio, cured meats, and sashimi (not sushi, though, because sushi has cooked rice). Sometimes I also call the restaurant ahead of time to see if they have alternatives that I can eat. If all else fails, I ask if they will sear my fish or meat—a little raw is better than none at all. I choose to put my health first—but it shouldn't mean missing out on social events or beating myself up if I'm not 100 percent. Life is not about perfection.

Carol's Tip

Bring your own salad dressing! You never know what's in restaurant salad dressings (I bet your waiter doesn't know either). Most of the time these dressings are bottled, not fresh, so they contain rancid, chemically processed oils and ingredients that make a healthy meal quickly become very unhealthy. Instead of relying on a restaurant to have fresh dressing, I carry my own mixture of cold-pressed olive oil and Udo's Choice Oil Blend in a little bottle and also bring my Power Organics salt. Or you can make your own homemade healthy salad topper and carry it in a little container (check out Dressing-2-Go containers online).

When I'm invited to parties, I often bring a platter of raw cheese and raw crackers for the host to serve. Most of the time people are very open and love trying new foods. It's always a big hit—people are often flabbergasted by how good everything tastes. Before I go to parties I also make sure I'm not hungry so I don't eat mindlessly. I find if I'm full, I'm less likely to eat garbage just because it's available.

Today there's so much amazing raw food out there that I never feel deprived. Dieting is about deprivation, while raw food is not. Once you dive into a raw lifestyle, you'll find that every word of that is true.

"WHAT ABOUT ALCOHOL?"

Technically, wine is considered raw. Unlike many other spirits, including hard alcohol and beer, wine is not distilled—which involves heating liquids to their boiling point. Wine is instead fermented over time.

I personally stay away from alcoholic beverages as much as possible. Eating raw is an overall lifestyle for me, and thanks to practitioners like Dr. Richard Firshein, the director and founder of the Firshein Center for Integrative Medicine in New York City, I've learned exactly what alcohol does to my liver. Don't get me wrong, I'm all about the occasional birthday or New Year's toast, but I'm always conscious about how much I drink.

Since alcohol is considered by many to be a critical part of any party or social gathering, I asked Dr. Firshein to explain the effects of alcohol on the liver:

> "The liver is the second-largest organ in our body and has the unique capacity to detoxify almost every biochemical process and toxin found in the body. If the substance is a toxin, such as alcohol, the liver will break it down and make it "biodegradable" so that it can be eliminated as waste. But that's up to a point—about 1 ounce of straight alcohol or a 4- to 6-ounce glass of wine or alcohol-diluted beverage.
>
> Because of the increasing amounts of toxins that we're constantly exposing ourselves to, our livers are completely overworked and overloaded. Once the liver's workload becomes more than it can handle, it creates a higher level of toxicity in the body, ultimately compromising your health. This happens quickly with alcohol, which the body can, in the case of wine, process at about 4 to 6 ounces per hour.

About 90 percent of all degenerative diseases can be traced to a dysfunctional or overstressed liver. Ultimately, this speeds up the aging process and contributes to the significant increase in cancers and chronic illnesses seen among heavy alcohol users. When these toxins are produced and/or not eliminated, they produce an acidic environment in the body that contributes to many diseases."

If you choose to indulge in an alcoholic drink, Dr. Firshein suggests an organic or biodynamic wine that is lower in sulfites, instead of a wine that uses sulfur dioxide as a preservative. Organic wine means fewer pesticides and chemical additives, which translates to lower toxicity and less stress on the liver. Many people experience intolerance or immune reactions to nonorganic alcohol. The symptoms could be anything from severe asthma, diarrhea, rashes, vomiting, runny nose, or swollen eyes in the short term to eczema, migraines, and chronic fatigue in the long term. So it's best to go organic when you can.

Remember, everything in moderation!

Carol's Tip

I find that when I have eaten enough during the day, I don't really need the sugar boost that alcohol gives me. Remember, I started my day with Scotch and coffee for seventeen years and was addicted to it! I broke that habit by feeding my body properly so that it didn't call for alcohol or sugar for a quick boost. When I do find myself craving alcohol, I take it as a signal that I have not nourished my body correctly that day.

Raw Recipes

One of the big myths about raw food that I would like to debunk is that a raw food diet is one of deprivation, where you can eat only rabbit food like lettuce and carrots. There are countless satisfying dishes that can be created by following the raw food guidelines. Nearly anything that you love can be created with raw foods, even ice cream! A raw diet (and actually any healthy diet) is all about planning and prepping. When you don't plan (which you will learn about more in "Grocery Shopping for Success," page 92), you will just grab and eat anything that is convenient. When I first started eating raw, every Sunday I would prep these four raw recipes and plop them in the refrigerator so that if I got hungry I could always make a meal or snack out of them.

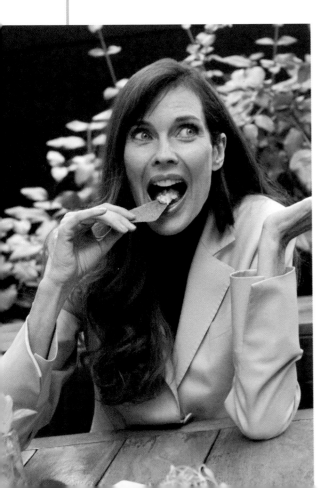

Salsa: Mix 2 cups chopped tomatoes, 1 tablespoon chopped red onion, and pinches of cilantro, salt, and cayenne pepper or ½ chopped jalapeño pepper (if you like spicy salsa).

Guacamole: Add 2 avocados to the salsa recipe and remove the jalapeño pepper.

Cucumber Salad: Thinly slice 1 large organic English cucumber. Dice half an onion and 1 avocado and combine with the cucumber. Mix 3 heaping table-spoons kefir with Udo's Choice cold-pressed extra-virgin olive oil and Celtic sea salt. Toss with the cucumber mix-ture and serve.

Lentil Salad: Dice 1 white onion, 1 tomato, and 1 organic English cucumber, and combine them with 1 cup raw, sprouted lentils (sprouts help the body absorb nutrients better). In a separate bowl, whisk 2 tablespoons Udo's Choice cold-pressed extra-virgin olive oil, 2 tablespoons raw apple cider vinegar, sea salt to taste, and juice from ¼ lemon. Add to the lentil mixture.

All these recipes take less than 5 minutes to prepare!

Don't stop there, though! I've reached out to some of my favorite raw foodies and bloggers for more delicious raw recipes to take you through your whole day! We've got you covered for every meal.

Carol's Tip

Keep snacks readily available! I always have good intentions and think "I'm not going to snack," but life happens—a friend stops by or I have a free night and watch TV—and snacks just add to the pleasure of the moment. There are plenty of raw snacks that last in the cupboard. I love dehydrated food!

BREAKFAST

Susan Powers at Rawmazing.com is revolutionizing the world of raw food cookery with her inventive and delicious recipes and beautiful food styling and photography. Susan is introducing the world to a whole new raw by bringing traditional food preparation methods into the raw world, and balancing flavor, color, texture, and mouthfeel.

RAW ORANGE-GINGER GLAZED DOUGHNUTS

By Susan Powers of Rawmazing, www.rawmazing.com

Makes 5 doughnuts*

2½ cups raw oat flour†
(made by grinding raw
flaked oats)

1 cup whole Brazil nuts,
ground fine

¼ cup raw, organic coconut
flour

1 teaspoon liquid stevia

⅓ cup coconut oil, melted

¼ cup coconut sugar

1 teaspoon cinnamon

1 teaspoon vanilla

1. Combine all ingredients in a large bowl.

2. To make doughnuts, press the dough firmly into a doughnut pan. Tip pan over and tap gently to release doughnuts.† Repeat until you've used all the dough.

3. Top with Orange-Ginger Glaze (recipe follows).

*This recipe makes 5 doughnuts, but due to the size, 1 doughnut should be considered 2 servings.

†Oat flours can differ greatly. If your dough is too dry, add a little moisture. Just note that you want to be able to press the doughnuts and mold them.

‡Alternatively, roll into 1½-inch balls and dip in the glaze.

Orange-Ginger Glaze

Zest from 1 orange

3 tablespoons orange juice

3 tablespoons raw coconut butter (not coconut oil), softened

6–9 drops liquid stevia

1 teaspoon grated fresh ginger

Whisk all ingredients together. Pour over doughnuts. Let set (this will take a couple of hours).

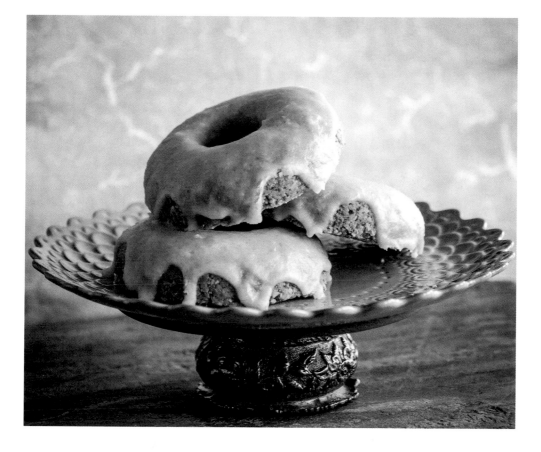

LUNCH

I recently sat down with Brad Gruno, whose company makes Brad's Raw Chips. These delicious chips are one of my favorite snacks! Brad was a construction worker who was a typical American guy. He was overweight, had high cholesterol and low energy, and didn't sleep well (sounds familiar!). He stumbled into raw food after a family member suggested it. He went 100 percent raw for the first year and says he'd never felt so good in his life. During this time, Brad wanted a crunchy snack and started experimenting with dehydrated kale chips, a discovery that led him to create Brad's Raw Chips. He started selling the chips at a local farmers' market, and eventually they grew into a national brand that is now available in a variety of flavors. Lucky for us, products like this have made becoming raw easier.

Brad's new raw cookbook, *Brad's Raw Made Easy,* further simplifies the raw lifestyle, and he was kind enough to share one of his favorite recipes with us.

AVOCADO SOUP

By Brad Gruno of Brad's Raw Foods

Makes 2 servings

1 avocado, sliced

¼ cup chopped spinach

¼ cup chopped red bell
   pepper

2 tablespoons diced red
   onion

1 clove garlic

1 tablespoon coconut oil, or
   to taste

¼ teaspoon ground cumin,
   or to taste

Diced jalapeño, to taste, plus
   more for garnish

Pinch of Himalayan sea salt,
   or to taste

Juice of ½ lime, plus wedges
   for garnish

Spring water

Brad's Raw Leafy Kale Nacho
   Chips, for garnish

1. Combine the avocado, spinach, bell pepper,
   red onion, garlic, coconut oil, cumin,
   jalapeño, and salt in a blender.

2. Squeeze in the lime juice.

3. Add spring water to halfway up the
   ingredients and blend until smooth.

4. Add more water until desired souplike
   consistency is reached.

5. Pour into bowls to serve.

6. Crush a handful of kale chips and sprinkle
   on the top.

7. Garnish with lime wedges and jalapeño.

8. Serve and enjoy!

DINNER

Sarma Melngailis is the cofounder of Pure Food and Wine, a raw food restaurant in New York City, and the founder and CEO of One Lucky Duck. Sarma is also the coauthor of *Raw Food/Real World* and the author of *Living Raw Food*.

ZUCCHINI AND HEIRLOOM TOMATO LASAGNA

By Sarma Melngailis, owner of Pure Food and Wine and One Lucky Duck in New York City

FOR "RICOTTA":

2 cups raw pine nuts, soaked in water for at least 1 hour

2 tablespoons lemon juice

2 tablespoons nutritional yeast

½ teaspoon sea salt

6 tablespoons filtered water

FOR TOMATO SAUCE:

2 cups sun-dried tomatoes, soaked in water for at least 2 hours

1 small to medium tomato, diced

¼ small onion, chopped

2 tablespoons lemon juice

2 tablespoons extra-virgin olive oil

1. To make the "ricotta": Combine the pine nuts, lemon juice, nutritional yeast, and salt in a food processor and pulse a few times until thoroughly blended. Gradually add the water and process for 1 to 2 minutes, until the texture becomes fluffy like ricotta.

2. To make the tomato sauce: Squeeze and drain as much water out of the sun-dried tomatoes as possible. Place in a food processor or high-speed blender with the remaining ingredients and blend until smooth.

3. To make the pesto: Place all the ingredients in a food processor and blend until well combined but still slightly chunky, 2 to 3 minutes.

½ teaspoon liquid stevia

1 teaspoon sea salt

Pinch of red pepper flakes

FOR PESTO:

2 cups packed fresh basil
leaves

½ cup raw pistachios

3 tablespoons extra-virgin
olive oil

½ teaspoon sea salt

Pinch of freshly ground black
pepper

FOR LASAGNA:

3 zucchini, halved crosswise
and thinly sliced
lengthwise

2 tablespoons extra-virgin
olive oil

1 tablespoon finely chopped
fresh oregano

1 tablespoon fresh thyme

Pinch of sea salt

Pinch of freshly ground black
pepper

3 heirloom tomatoes, halved
and sliced

Whole basil leaves, for
garnish

4. To assemble the lasagna: Toss the zucchini with the olive oil, oregano, thyme, salt, and pepper. Place 3 zucchini slices, slightly overlapping, in the center of each serving plate to make a square shape. Spread the tomato sauce over the zucchini, top with small dollops of "ricotta" and pesto, and add a few tomato slices. Repeat twice more, creating three layers in total per serving. Garnish with basil leaves.

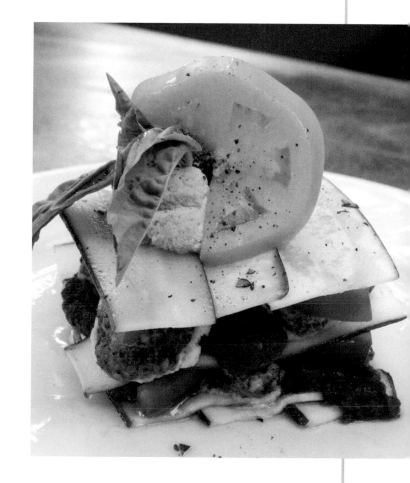

DESSERT

Gena Hamshaw is a certified clinical nutritionist and author of the blog *Choosing Raw* and a cookbook by the same name. Her work has been published in *O, The Oprah Magazine* and *VegNews* magazine and on the websites Food52 and Whole Living Daily. She sees clients around the country, and specializes in digestive health, disordered-eating histories, and plant-based diets.

RAW VEGAN BLACKBERRY CHEESECAKE BARS

By Gena Hamshaw of Choosing Raw, www.choosingraw.com

Makes 15 to 20 bars, depending on how big you'd like them

1½ cups walnuts

1 cup pitted dates

¼ teaspoon sea salt, divided

1 cup cashews, soaked in
water for at least 2 hours
and drained

1 cup blackberries

½ cup melted coconut oil

⅓ cup maple syrup*

* Dr. Perlmutter recommends using
1 teaspoon of liquid stevia instead
of maple syrup.

1. Lightly grease a 7 × 11-inch baking pan or casserole dish with olive or coconut oil.

2. To make the bottom layer, place the walnuts, dates, and ⅛ teaspoon of the sea salt in a food processor and pulse to break the ingredients down until they're crumbled. Process until the mixture is ground up and sticks together when you squeeze some in your hand.

3. Press the mixture into the prepared baking pan and set aside (or chill overnight if making ahead).

4. To make the top layer, blend the cashews, blackberries, coconut oil, the remaining ⅛ teaspoon sea salt, and the maple syrup in a high-speed blender or food processor and process until the mixture is as smooth as possible. Pour into the pan over the prepared bottom layer. Use a spatula to spread the top layer evenly.

5. Chill for at least 3 hours. Cut into bars and serve.

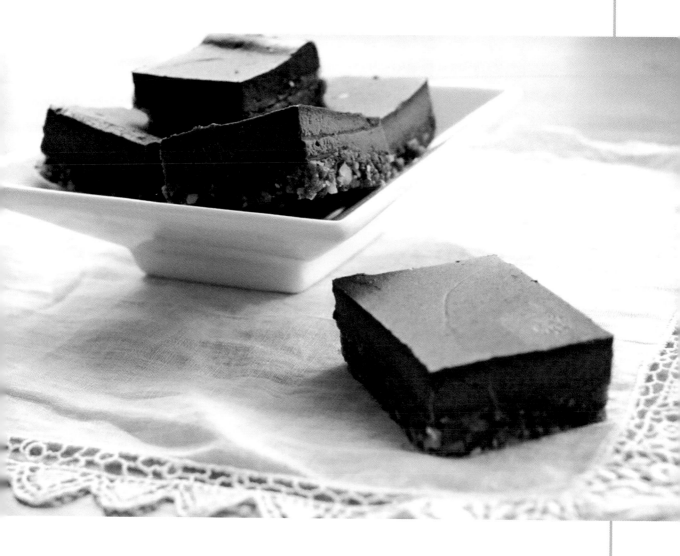

Steps in the Raw Direction

If a raw diet *still* sounds like too much for you to commit to, you can start out by replacing your favorite snacks with healthier alternatives. Every one of these steps is in the right direction! I asked Liana Werner-Gray, author of *The Earth Diet*, which chronicles her journey to health after she was diagnosed with a precancerous tumor, to share some suggestions on integrating raw food into your life (including her favorite healthy sweet snack!):

Junk: Most snack chips contain chemicals and genetically modified ingredients that have no nutritional value.

Replace with: Kale chips or vegetable chips made from beets or zucchini. (You can make your own crispy treats by placing kale on a baking sheet with a sprinkle of nutritional yeast and salt, and baking it at 115°F for 15 minutes.)

Junk: Soda is highly acidic and the diet versions often contain aspartame, a sweetener that is linked to cancer, diabetes, and depression.

Replace with: Raw coconut water or KeVita, a probiotic drink that's sweet and fizzy, just like soda!

Carol's Tip

Try replacing energy drinks with Xocai, a raw energy drink. I introduced Bill O'Reilly to this great alternative!

Junk: Candy provides the body no nutrients and creates a blood sugar spike.

Replace with: Fruit leather. This healthy alternative is essentially just fruit that has a texture similar to candy. Make your own by pureeing apples, pears, or any fruit you want in a blender. Then spread the puree on a parchment-lined baking sheet and bake for 7½ hours at 115°F (or until it reaches a consistency that pleases you), or use a food dehydrator, then cut the dried puree into strips. They will be like a gummy candy. You can also buy fruit leather at the store, but making it yourself allows you to control the ingredients.

Junk: Most cookies are highly processed and made from refined flours and sugar. They cause digestion issues because they are loaded with gluten and are very hard for the body to process.

Replace with: Raw cookie dough! This is by far one of Liana's most popular recipes. It is essentially made with three ingredients: almond flour (made only from ground almonds, it's gluten-free) or nut meal, honey, and some vanilla. These three ingredients make a delicious cookie dough flavor! You can add a dash of evaporated sea salt or Himalayan salt and throw in some nut pieces or cacao nibs to make a chocolate chip flavor! The cookie dough takes 5 minutes to make and is ready to eat right away. If you eat it raw you will get a big dose of nutrients, especially antioxidants and protein. And watch out: it will fill you up in a hurry!

RAW ALMOND "CHOCOLATE CHIP" COOKIE DOUGH BALLS

By Liana Werner-Gray

Makes 12 balls

2 cups almond meal or flour

1 teaspoon pure vanilla extract

3 large, soft dates, mashed

¼ teaspoon salt

2 tablespoons cacao nibs

1. Combine the almond meal, vanilla, mashed dates, and salt in a large bowl. Once the mixture is well blended, stir in the cacao nibs.

2. Taste and add more dates if you would like the dough to be sweeter. It should be moist enough to hold together; add water if needed.

3. Roll the dough into ½-inch balls and serve.

4. Store leftover dough balls—if there are any—in the fridge for up to 3 weeks. In the freezer they will stay good for up to 2 months.

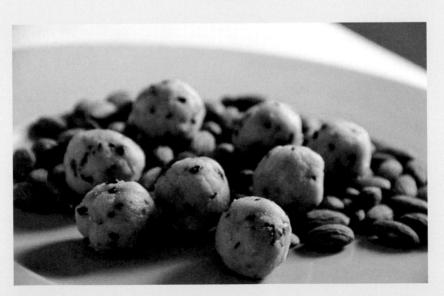

TIPS:

- If you want to bake the dough balls, bake at 200°F for 1 hour.
- To keep them raw, dehydrate them by baking at 115°F for 4 hours.
- Use a vanilla bean if possible. Scrape the seeds from the bean pod and add them where vanilla is called for in the recipe. If using vanilla extract, choose one without added sugar—check the ingredients on the label.
- You can make this recipe without the cacao nibs, but the nibs are what make it "chocolate chip."

VARIATIONS:

- **Peanut Butter Cookie Dough Balls:** Add 3 tablespoons peanut butter to the dough mixture.
- **Chocolate Cookie Dough Balls:** Add 1 tablespoon cacao powder to the dough mixture.
- **Chocolate-Covered Cookie Dough Balls:** On a plate, roll the balls in 1½ tablespoons cacao powder.

BENEFITS:

- High in protein
- Gluten-free
- Vegan
- High in antioxidants
- Brain food
- High in magnesium, which relaxes the muscles
- Can be used as an antidepressant
- Increases energy
- Replaces processed cookie cravings

Eat more real food and skip the processed foods—*you can do this!*

Ask Carol

If you can't always eat real foods, what are some of your favorite packaged raw items that can be purchased in a grocery store?

ANSWER:

- KeVita (probiotic drink): my favorite flavor is lemon ginger!

- Raw Revolution: bars

- Udo's Choice: oils for use in salads

- Go Raw: granola and bars

- Two Moms in the Raw: truffles

- Nature's Fuel Raw Bars: my favorite flavor is Rocky Road!

- Organic Food Bars

- Greens+ Natural Energy Bars

- Raw nuts, seeds, and dried fruit

- Raw milk cheese

Carol's Tip

Every product and recipe mentioned in this book is here because I
have interviewed the experts or love their food. You are getting what I
love and what I have found that works!

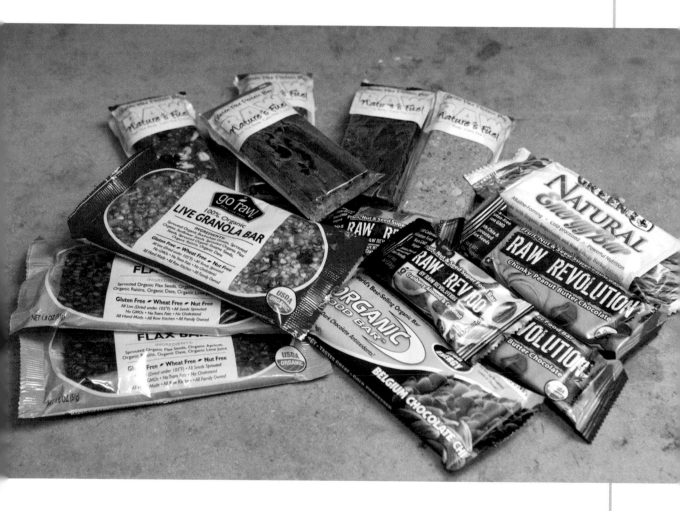

"Which Diet Is the Best for Me?"

Every week it seems like there's a new diet or eating program on the market or in the news. It becomes all the rage for a while and then quickly fizzles out. How are we supposed to know which one is the best for our health? Should you be vegan, raw, vegetarian, Paleo, carnivore, or clean eating? Should you eat for your blood type or your feelings about animals? What about the Seasonal Diet, Grapefruit Diet, or Mediterranean Diet? With all the information out there, all the programs, all the studies, it's no wonder people are confused.

I spoke to my go-to doctor in New York City, Nicholas Gonzalez, MD, to find an answer. Dr. Gonzalez is a physician specializing in alternative treatments that are based on the belief that pancreatic enzymes, supplements, and detox are among the body's main defenses against cancer and other diseases.

Dr. Gonzalez agreed that there is a lot of conflicting evidence about what humans should eat. "Each book contradicts the previous book, people end up more confused than when they started, and often end up not feeling any better." I couldn't agree more! Before I discovered that a raw diet was for me, I would get caught up in each new trend, always hoping for a quick fix. According to Dr. Gonzalez, "Humans are a very variable species and have occupied just about every ecological niche around the world." Everyone is different and should eat how their particular ancestors ate.

"Food is fuel and you have to put the right fuel into the right engine. If you put water into a Mercedes-Benz, you have just ruined your car, and if you put diesel fuel into a steam engine, it's going to explode. You need to tailor what you eat to the way your ancestors ate."

Dr. Gonzalez follows the research of Dr. Weston Price, who traveled the world searching for isolated cultural groups who still followed their traditional lifestyle and diet. His journeys took him from the Eskimos in the Arctic to the Inca descendants in the high Andes, to the Masai in the plains of Kenya and the peoples in the high Swiss Alpine valleys and the faraway Polynesian islands. His findings can be summed up in one basic principle: depending on where we're located, our species has adapted to, and appears to thrive on, quite different diets that often seem to have little in common. And to Price's surprise, in the case of the people he studied, as varied as each diet was, each group seemed to enjoy excellent good health, free from degenerative diseases such as allergies, arthritis, cancer, diabetes, heart disease, and even mental illness to some extent.

For example, though the specifics may vary depending on whether they're near the sea or farther inland, Eskimos have long consumed a diet consisting primarily of red meat from caribou and water mammals, such as seals and walrus, and almost no fruits or vegetables. Their diet has been very high in saturated fat, yet they are healthy. Over generations, their bodies have adapted to this type of food intake. Eskimo populations didn't experience high rates of diseases like cancer until they moved to Western villages and adopted Western-style eating patterns that included bread and other heavily processed products.

Another example: if you're of Northern European ancestry, you can probably digest milk, and if you're Southeast Asian, you probably can't. In most mammals, the gene for lactose tolerance switches off once an animal matures beyond the weaning years. Humans shared that fate as well—until a mutation in the DNA of an isolated population of Northern Europeans around ten thousand years ago introduced an adaptive tolerance for nutrient-rich milk. The likelihood that you can tolerate milk depends on the degree to which you have Northern European blood.

But wait? America's a melting pot! What does this mean for us?

I'll let Dr. Gonzalez explain.

How to Eat Like Our Ancestors

By Dr. Nicholas Gonzalez, MD

Modern Americans couldn't differ more greatly from isolated peoples, as America is inhabited and built by people from all continents and cultures, whose ancestors adapted to a variety of diets. So how do we adapt Price's principles and choose a diet suited to our ancestral background? Actually, as complicated and bewildering as such determinations might seem, it really isn't that difficult. I learned a long time ago that people tend to need, for optimal biological effect, the very foods that they like, that they even crave. Sounds simple, but it really, really works in practice.

If we look at other species for a moment, carnivores, such as lions, like to eat meat. They choose meat, because it's what they are designed for and the food they use efficiently. No self-respecting lion would ever think about munching on grass, or on leaves, or on hay. They want meat. But a natural vegetarian like a gazelle, for instance, chooses and thrives on grass and greens, on plants, and will never opt to eat meat, like a rabbit, ever.

We should follow this lead from nature. Humans, such as Eskimos, who are genetically programmed to require meat *like* meat. They don't want grains, salads, or even fruit particularly, though they might force themselves to consume these plant foods because they are so heavily promoted as "healthy" in books and the media. Despite popular misconceptions, genetic meat eaters should be eating meat, the fattier the better, as much as desired, forgetting the leafy greens and the fruit. They should eat as much fat—the Eskimo diet was high fat and high protein—as they want.

Of course in our practice rarely do we prescribe *just* meat: we find most of our "carnivore" patients do well with certain plant foods such as root vegetables like potatoes and sweet potatoes, as well as cruciferous vegetables like broccoli.

Our vegetarian patients will gag at the thought of bacon or pot roast, and so will find a salad for lunch with some beans, nuts, and dressing quite sufficient for their appetites, and to keep up their stamina the rest of the afternoon. They want to eat light, they like to eat plants, and only occasionally will they indulge in some lean fish or poultry.

Balanced people—balanced in terms of dietary needs—fall somewhere in between the vegetarians and the carnivores, functioning best with both plant foods, including fruits, vegetables, grains, nuts, seeds, and beans, and some animal products, though not as much as our dedicated carnivores require. Such folks, who really want to eat a variety of foods, do well at a buffet providing a host of different eating possibilities.

People feel best when they provide the right fuel—that is, the right food—for their bodies and feel less well when they eat the wrong foods, take in the wrong fuel. That's a simple thought, but in practice it works. If you crave a certain type of food, you most likely need it. The brain knows what we should be doing and eating—after all, it has our best interests at heart. It's the experts that confuse and confound. Just try to make smart choices when you crave something sweet—go for a healthy real sweetness like raw cacao or fruit instead of a candy bar.

So whatever the experts say, your brain is smarter than they are. Learn to trust your inclinations, and your brain will lead you in the right direction, to the right food, and to the potential for lasting good health.

My Top Tips Everyone Can Follow

1. **Eat real food.** Fresh, whole, unrefined, and unprocessed food. Like what our ancestors ate! Eat as close to nature as possible because the further removed food is from its source, the less good "data" it will contain.

2. **Don't calorie count.** Calories really don't matter as much as what nutrients are in the food. Coconut oil may be caloric, but it is also loaded with benefits from its nutrients and may actually help you lose weight.

3. **Eat a wide variety of food.** Conversely, don't overload on just one food or one type of fat. For example, I had someone write me that after reading my first book, she gained weight, and she wanted to know why that happened if she had followed the guidance in my book. After several emails, she confessed that she loved the avocado sandwich and ate three or four a day! No wonder she gained weight. She was eating far too much of one food.

4. **Enjoy your food and take your time eating it,** preferably in the company of people you love.

5. **Prepare your own meals.**

6. **Don't waste your time feeling guilty if you ate the "wrong" thing.** Instead, have a bottle of digestive enzymes on hand and take a few to give your digestive tract some assistance.

   Digestive enzymes aid in the absorption of vitamins and minerals and assist in breaking down the food you eat. This process allows the food to be used as energy, which supports the building of new muscle and nerve cells and protects your blood from toxins. Inadequate enzyme production can lead to digestive discomfort, gas, bloating, low energy, and allergy-like reactions to food. And for your next meal, try to eat better!

Food Allergies and Intolerances

OK, so now you get it. It's important for everyone to go back to nature and eat real, unprocessed food. But sometimes that still isn't enough to feel your very best. What happens when you eat real foods but still feel sluggish, bloated, or groggy afterward? Or perhaps you have more severe symptoms like nausea or diarrhea after a meal?

You might have a food allergy or intolerance. It's important to be in tune with your body and be able to tell when it reacts improperly to certain types of foods. I know what you are thinking: Carol, it's worth it for me to have an upset stomach after pizza—I love it! Well, that might justify the uneasiness this week or this year. But where the real problem lies is in the long term. If left untreated, this simple stomachache can lead to major digestive issues, sleep problems, sinus infections, obesity, premature aging, or even anaphylaxis (an allergic shock that can result in death). You might even be suffering from one or two of these issues right now and never thought to connect it to a food allergy. This was true in my case!

Before I went raw I had terrible sinus issues. I never left my home without nasal spray or sinus and allergy medication because I was in severe pain without them. They ran my life. I remember being on film sets and having anxiety that I would leave my medicine in a coat pocket and not be able to sleep during the night. My whole day revolved around easy access to my medication. Eventually things got so bad that I went to an ear, nose, and throat doctor because I needed to figure out what was going on. He suggested I get nasal surgery and allow him to cut into my sinuses. Thank God I didn't let him do it. I knew surgery wasn't the answer and that there had to be another way.

When I went raw, I stopped eating gluten—pasta, bagels and bread, pizza, and so on. As another wonderful side effect, besides all the other things going raw did for me, my sinuses cleared up immediately. Immediately! Not a week later, not a month later; literally from the moment I eliminated gluten from my diet, I felt better.

As it turns out, I have had an undiagnosed food allergy to gluten since I was a child. This allergy and its debilitating side effects had built up in my system from my unknowingly devouring gluten for all those years. By my twenties, it had already manifested itself as a bad sinus problem. But I never thought to connect my sinus issues with the food I was eating.

Like many of you, I never thought I could give up wheat—at the time I was eating bread, pasta, and other wheat products all day long. Going raw made me realize that feeling good every day was far more important than the immediate satisfaction I got from eating pizza. Yes, it's delicious, and I still do indulge once in a while, but overall I know my body is healthier without it. That was seventeen years ago now and I'm still clear about that.

Before we get too far along here, there is an important distinction that needs to be made between food allergies and food "sensitivities," which can be problematic but usually not as severe.

I sat down with Dr. Vincent Giampapa, a leader in the field of anti-aging, who offered some useful suggestions for navigating this world of allergies and sensitivities to food. I met Dr. Giampapa in an airport lounge after I accidentally missed my flight—again I believe everything happens for a reason! Dr. Giampapa began his work as a means of rectifying his own allergies, as he found out, to such vegetables as spinach and kale.

First he explained to me the difference between allergies and sensitivities.

WHAT IS A FOOD ALLERGY?

A food allergy is often diagnosed when you are young, but, as with my allergy, this is not always the case. Sometimes it can build up undetected inside your system. An allergy is your immune system's response to the food you have recently eaten. Your body mistakes an ingredient, usually a protein, as harmful and creates a defense system (antibodies) to fight it. An allergic reaction occurs when the antibodies are battling an "invading" food protein, and it affects numerous organs in the body. Food allergies can be severe, so if you believe you have one of the symptoms described below, please contact your doctor immediately, as an allergy can lead to closing of the throat, severe sickness, or even anaphylactic shock and death.

The most common foods that cause allergic reactions are:

- Eggs

- Fish

- Peanuts

- Milk

- Nuts from trees (Brazil nuts, walnuts, almonds, and hazelnuts)

- Shellfish

- Gluten

- Wine

WHAT ARE THE SYMPTOMS OF A FOOD ALLERGY?

Symptoms of a food allergy can range from mild to severe, and the amount of food necessary to trigger a reaction varies from person to person. Symptoms include:

- Rash or hives
- Nausea
- Cramping stomach pain
- Diarrhea
- Itchy skin
- Sinus infection
- Runny nose
- Chest pain
- Swelling of the airways to the lungs

WHAT IS FOOD INTOLERANCE?

A food intolerance is a digestive system response rather than an immune system response that occurs when food irritates a person's digestive system or when a person is unable to properly digest, or break down, food because of an enzyme deficiency. It happens immediately or a few days after certain foods are eaten.

When you struggle with bloating, gas, indigestion, and other bowel problems for too many years, your intestinal lining will become irritated and inflamed. This compromises your digestion and overall health, and if these issues go on for years, they can weaken the immune system, which leads to disease. Fifty percent of our immune system is found in our digestive tract so we want everything there to be functioning at an optimal level.

The most common foods that cause intolerance are:

- Beans
- Cabbage
- Citrus fruit
- Grains
- Milk (lactose)
- Processed meats

WHAT ARE THE SYMPTOMS OF FOOD INTOLERANCE?

- Nausea
- Stomach pain
- Gas, cramps, or bloating
- Vomiting
- Heartburn
- Diarrhea
- Headaches
- Irritability or nervousness

Food intolerances can also manifest with milder and nonspecific symptoms, such as eczema, concentration and learning difficulties, hyperactivity, poor sleep, irritability or mood swings, low energy, and so on.

It's easy to see why people often confuse food allergies and food intolerances because they have similar symptoms. The key points to remember are:

Food allergy = Immune system response
Food intolerance = Digestive system response

It is vital that you begin to pay attention to your body, if you are not already doing so, to get in tune with it so you can tell if you have any of these symptoms, identify the culprit food with a trained allergist, and treat the problem.

To help figure out if you have an allergy, Dr. Giampapa suggests, talk to your doctor and take an ALCAT (antigen leukocyte antibody test). The ALCAT is a lab-based immune stimulation test in which a patient's white blood cells are challenged with various substances, including foods, additives, colorings, chemicals, medicinal herbs, functional foods, molds, and pharmaceutical compounds. Each patient has a unique set of responses that helps to identify the potentially harmful trigger substances.

If you want to treat without a test, you can try a two-week elimination diet. Eliminate one food or food group at a time. Animal milk and dairy products, wheat and gluten, eggs, and coffee are probably the most common foods that cause intolerance problems, but any food can be a problem, so be open-minded. Foods will need to be avoided strictly for an initial two-week period. If your symptoms improve significantly during this time, the eliminated food may be responsible for the reactions.

After you've identified the culprit, Dr. Giampapa suggests eliminating this food from your diet.

Restoring Your Gut

I had Dr. Robert Scott Bell, who suffered from allergies throughout his childhood, on my show to discuss his experience with allergies. He surprised everyone by saying, "Your allergies are not causing your stuffy nose."

He explained that an allergy is a hypersensitivity of the immune system and, while it can sometimes be described as an acute reaction, it's really a chronic underlying problem with your gut.

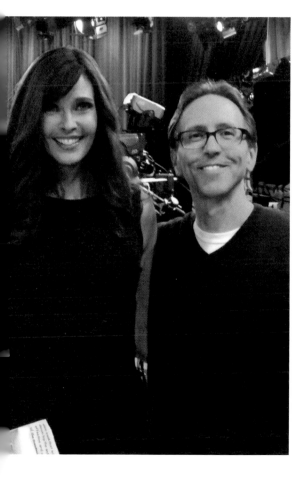

I'll let Dr. Bell take it from here:

"The first mistake most Americans make when trying to relieve their allergies is to suppress the allergic symptoms while ignoring the underlying factors that brought them about. While you may feel better temporarily on a drugstore medication, you run the risk of making the underlying condition much worse.

But what is that condition? The health of your gut!

Allergies start long before you actually notice that you have them, often because of damage to the gastrointestinal lining in childhood from well-meaning doctors prescribing antibiotics. These anti-bacterial drugs can be life-saving in serious situations, but they indiscriminately kill the vital healthy flora lining your stomach and colon, too.

That would be bad enough, but in the process of killing the bugs, the lining of the gastrointestinal tract is left damaged and inflamed. The gut, once teeming with beneficial bacterial life-forms, is now left desolate, like a sandy desert with occasional pools of quicksand. When this occurs, undigested protein macromolecules can cross a now-permeable gut barrier, just as sure as microbes have easy access to your blood should you have an open wound on your skin.

Pathogenic bacteria, viruses, and even fungal species like *Candida albicans* can take advantage of such a damaged state as well. They would normally not have access to the bloodstream, but when the gut lining is compromised, the gate openings become large enough for access to formerly prohibited substances and life-forms. When undigested proteins enter the bloodstream, they elicit powerful immune responses appropriate to repelling the intruders."

This damaged state from a lack of probiotics can go undetected, often for years. The immune system is always on, always responding to this incursion with each and every meal. When the immune system is constantly in reactionary mode, it begins to hyper-respond or hyper-react to normally occurring substances in the environment as well—pump up that antihistamine.

Yet we wrongly blame the allergens. Dust, mold, animal dander, grasses, pollen, weed, dairy, grain—you pick one or all of them. I was the poster child for pretty much all of them in my young life. While the trigger may vary from person to person, the stage was set deep inside the body well before it first manifested as an allergy. All the over-the-counter and prescription drugs and allergy shots did little besides manage symptoms. They never addressed the underlying chronic gut inflammation.

Since most doctors are trained to only manage symptoms, you will rarely find an allergist who focuses on restoring gut integrity in order to ultimately rid you of your allergies. I do not mean to oversimplify the process of healing, nor downplay your desire for symptomatic relief. You can actually achieve both.

Homeopathic remedies such as *Allium cepa, Sticta pulmonaria,* and *Kali bichromicum* are often successful at minimizing symptom severity, particularly when the sinuses are involved. Since Latin-named homeopathic single remedies are often confusing or intimidating for someone new to homeopathy, complex formulations for many different types of allergies are available from King Bio to make symptom management, including for regional allergies, much easier (and safer, since there are no side effects). I am often met with much gratitude from those who I have introduced to silver hydrosol for spraying directly into the sinuses as well. The silver works as an astringent, cleansing the area of allergen triggers, while reducing tissue inflammation as well.

More important, the correction happens deeper in the GI tract with a focus on restoring epithelial integrity to the gut lining, including enzyme and probiotic restoration. And remember to take a good probiotic each and every day.

Carol's Tip

Colloidal silver (silver hydrosol) is also great for sore throats!

Ask Carol

I have a gluten allergy and have tried to eliminate gluten from my diet (eating all gluten-free foods!).
Why do I still feel sick?

ANSWER:

I'm going to turn to Jennifer Esposito to answer this one!

Jennifer, an actress and the owner of Jennifer's Way, a gluten-free bakery in New York City, was diagnosed with celiac disease, an autoimmune disorder characterized by a severe reaction to gluten. Like you, she ate gluten-free foods and was confused by the fact that she was still not feeling well. After doing research and working with Dr. Patrick Fratellone, Jennifer realized that not all gluten-free foods are created equal—some products claim to be gluten-free but still contain some gluten. Also, gluten isn't only in wheat-based items, it's present in products where you least expect it like soup, fillers, vinegar, certain tea bags, and even hair and beauty products. If you have celiac disease, you need to do a full house and food overhaul. For more information check out Jennifer's book *Jennifer's Way* or JennifersWay.org.

Understanding Fats

Now that you've learned that you need to eat real foods and be more aware of how what you eat affects your body, you've probably decided you're going to eat healthier. Good for you! One of the first things many people do as they set out to eat better is avoid fat. But the truth is, your body needs fat to function properly.

In fact, way back in 1929, George and Mildred Burr, a husband-and-wife research team, discovered that omega-6 fats were actually essential for health. This was first determined by working with rats that were put on a strictly fat-free diet and then reintroduced to fat after the researchers had documented the negative effects of fat deficiency. (The Burrs used a commonly available omega-6 fat. The health benefits of omega-3 fats were discovered in the 1980s.) Based on their important work with the rats, the Burrs subsequently coined the term "essential fatty acids."

Prior to their research, the common belief—and misunderstanding—was that all fatty acids could be synthesized from dietary carbohydrates. Because of the Burrs' initial findings and the discoveries that have been made since, we now know that omega-3s and omega-6s, the two essential fatty acids (or EFAs), are key to good health.

Even though the essentiality of omega-6 was proven long ago, the low-fat craze took the United States by storm in the early 1980s, and still remains a popular diet strategy for many people. People were told that eating fat-free foods was the secret to better health. Ads in grocery stores trumpeted fat-free and low-fat foods and snacks. These foods were everywhere and, amazingly, still are today! Thankfully, over time information about the importance of omega-3 and omega-6 EFAs has spread, and the low-fat trend has slowed down some. But many people are still indoctrinated with the idea that all fats are bad—something that couldn't be further from the truth!

Now that we have mostly recovered from the fat-free diet fad, which in the end was a big fat mistake, we have learned three important things:

1. The fat-free food we thought was so good for our health was very often filled with sugar and other carbohydrates. What many people don't understand is that the body turns excess sugar and other carbohydrates into fats (not the good kind), which is why we call carbohydrates the "undeclared fats."

2. Not all fats are created equal: different types of dietary fat play different roles in health and nutrition.

3. Through education, we can understand the critical difference between good and bad fats, and how to put that knowledge into practice to improve our health.

Let's go over the basics. There are two main kinds of fats:

1. **Essential fats,** both of which are polyunsaturated:

   - **Omega-3 fats** (3 double bonds or more): Essential alphalinolenic acid (ALA) and derivatives (EPA, DHA, and others). These fats are abundantly found in flax and chia seeds. Omega-3 derivatives are found in krill, mussels, and fish. These fats are liquid at room temperature.

   - **Omega-6 fats** (2 double bonds or more): Essential linoleic acid (LA) and derivatives (GLA, ARA, and others). Rich sources include sunflower, grapeseed, and corn oils, but all seeds and nuts contain them. Omega-6 derivatives are found in evening primrose oil, as well as in animal products. These fats are liquid at room temperature.

2. Nonessential fats:

- **Monounsaturated fats** (1 double bond): Rich sources include olives and olive oil, avocados, high-oleic sunflower or safflower oil, and almond, peanut, corn, sesame, rice bran, soybean, and cod liver oils. These fats are liquid at room temperature.

- **Saturated fats** (no double bonds): Rich sources include butter, lard, cheese, and meats like beef, lamb, and pork, but they are also found in tropical plant fats like coconut oil and palm oil. Saturated fats raise total blood and low-density lipoprotein (LDL) cholesterol levels, and can increase risk of cardiovascular disease and type 2 diabetes. These fats are solid at room temperature.

Omega-3s and omega-6s are defined as essential for the following reasons:

- They are a necessary component of cell membranes and are required for normal cell, tissue, gland, and organ functions, all of which are necessary for basic human health and functioning.

- The body cannot make EFAs from any other nutrient and therefore must get them directly from edible oils, whole foods, or oil supplements containing them.

- If you don't consume enough EFAs, deficiency symptoms start to show. Not getting enough for a long enough time can lead to death.

- Optimizing your intake of EFAs reverses the health problems and symptoms that come from deficiencies.

So, what happens when you don't get enough of these essential fatty acids? Because EFAs are required by every part of your body—cells, tissue, glands, and organs—to function properly, the signs of deficiency are many and bodywide, including:

- Low energy levels
- Deterioration of liver and kidneys
- Decreased ability to cope with stress and other behavioral changes
- Immune system deterioration, resulting in more infections, poorer wound healing, and increased risk for cancer
- Digestion problems, inflammation, bloating, allergies, autoimmune conditions
- Bone mineral loss
- Reproductive failure: sterility in males and miscarriage in females
- Developmental problems for children

- Tingling in arms and legs due to nerve deterioration
- Vision and learning problems
- Insulin resistance
- Increased risk of being overweight
- Increased cardiovascular risk
- In mental illness, increased symptoms
- Decreased lung function
- Decreased tissue oxidation
- Brittle hair and hair loss
- Poor nail growth
- Dry skin
- Constipation

The best way to oil our skin is from within. Since the body can survive with dry skin, its natural intelligence dictates that skin gets oils last and loses them first. Dry skin is an excellent indicator as to whether you are getting enough good dietary fats. This shows up as leathery, prematurely wrinkled, dry, or even scaly skin, and is more apparent during winter and in drier climates. To help my skin stay healthy, in addition to eating oils, I also rub raw fats such as olive oil and coconut oil on my face.

I spoke with Dr. Udo Erasmus, author of *Fats That Heal, Fats That Kill,* to better understand the difference between healthy and unhealthy fats and oils. He explained, "Good oils—especially the essential ones—

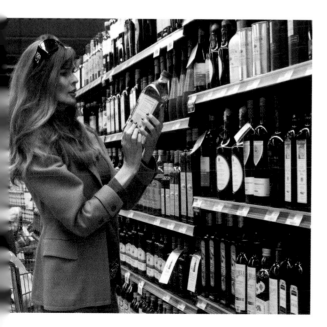

are easily damaged by heat, light, and oxygen, which is why it is so important to take care of them. More health problems come from damaged oils than any other part of nutrition. The health problems that we blame on oils should be blamed on the destructive industrial processing and cooking damage to which oils are commonly subjected. This is the crucial difference between the fats that heal and the fats that kill."

What turns a good fat bad? The short answer, according to Dr. Erasmus: processing and food preparation. Here's his longer answer:

1. Harsh Industrial Processing

- **Processed oils and foods that contain them:** When we treat plant-based cooking and salad oils with harsh chemicals and overheat them at frying temperatures, about 1 percent of the molecules change from being natural and good for the body to being unnatural and bad for it. In just 1 tablespoon of such an oil, we get more than one million damaged oil molecules for every one of our body's 60 trillion cells. That's the unstated reason why many health practitioners recommend not using oils at all; they don't make a distinction between good oils made with health in mind and bad oils damaged by processing. Making that distinction is really important for your health.

  Before 1986, when healthier oils became more readily available, the most common plant-based cooking and salad oils were damaged. These oils included all of the colorless, odorless, tasteless oils stored at room temperature in stores (except for those labeled "unrefined"), including corn, sunflower, safflower, cottonseed, soybean, walnut, sesame, almond, peanut, and rapeseed (canola) oils. These oils were also added to many hyperprocessed foods, including margarines and shortenings.

  The damaging refining processes to which most of these nonorganic oils were subjected helped manufacturers make perishable oils shelf stable for years or made liquid oils solid. These vegetable oils introduced a lot of toxic omega-6 molecules as well as pesticides into the food supply and our bodies.

When we began to cook our foods in oils instead of water, we made an already bad situation a whole lot worse.

- **Partial hydrogenation:** This destructive process turns cheap vegetable oils into solid, spreadable (plastic), shelf-stable, partially hydrogenated vegetable oils that contain trans-fatty acids. According to the Harvard School of Public Health, trans fats double the risk for a heart attack, interfere with immune function, and affect vision and learning development in children. Trans fats are associated with degenerative diseases that kill 68 percent of Western populations.

  Trans fats are found in margarines and shortenings (sometimes listed as vegetable shortening), and many processed commercial foods: cakes, pies, cookies, airplane foods, doughnuts, crackers, chips, pretzels, movie theater and microwaveable popcorn, frozen pizzas, coffee creamers, and salad dressings, to name some products. Even dried raisins and cranberries can be covered with them. The most effective way to avoid trans fats is to avoid processed foods. Instead, eat raw or prepare your own food using fresh organic ingredients. And read food labels—food manufacturers are required to list trans fats on the labels of products that contain them.

2. Cooking and Food-Preparation Habits

Frying, sautéing, roasting, and any other high-heat cooking method turns an otherwise good fat into a bad one. Research consistently shows that fried fats correlate with increased risk of cancer and cardiovascular problems. While frying temperatures damage even stable saturated fats such as butter, the more unsaturated the oil, the more toxic it becomes from high-heat cooking. Frying is, hands down, the single most destructive cooking method invented by humans: it damages our food and turns good fats into killer fats.

SO WHY IS THE RATIO OF OMEGA-3s TO OMEGA-6s SO IMPORTANT?

In today's Western diet, excessive amounts of omega-6 fatty acids are found in the food supply, with a very high average ratio of about 1:18 omega-3s to omega-6s. Ninety-nine percent of the population is deficient in omega-3 fatty acids. Cheap and overused vegetable oils contain high levels of omega-6s, and they and the hyperprocessed foods they are found in are the main culprits behind the imbalance in the Western diet.

What is the ideal ratio? We know for sure that we consume too many unhealthy omega-6s and too little omega-3s, and that the balance of omega-3 and omega-6 fatty acids is important for a stable, regular internal environment, and for normal development throughout the life cycle.

In almost thirty years of practice, working with thousands of people in more than thirty countries, Dr. Erasmus has found that a 2:1 ratio (a higher intake of omega-3s than omega-6s) addresses the imbalance and consistently gets the best results. He calls this the "practical" ratio: it's what works best, in practice, for optimal health.

Dr. Erasmus also recommends consuming 2 to 4 tablespoons of healthy oils per day (or about 1 tablespoon per fifty pounds of body weight) mixed into foods and spread out over the course of the day. Healthy oils include unrefined coconut oils, cold-pressed olive oil, or Udo's Choice, which contains seed and nut oils. These two basic recommendations alone address the need for optimal amounts of undamaged essential omega-3s and omega-6s, as well as correct the harmful imbalance of eating too many omega-6s.

Now that we understand the basics of good fats and bad fats, how do we turn this knowledge into practice?

1. Avoid damaged supermarket oils (the ones in clear plastic bottles, unrefrigerated) and the many processed foods that contain them. Learn to read labels and avoid foods containing ingredients such as "partially hydrogenated" oil and "trans-fatty acids." Note: "Zero trans-fatty acids" on a label actually means that the product can contain up to 0.5 percent of trans fats. "Zero" doesn't mean zero in this case!

2. Limit your intake of saturated fats. Unless it's raw cheese, dairy, or butter, lower your intake of hard fats like butter, lard, shortening, and margarine, and the fat in beef, dairy, cheese, lamb, and pork.

3. Choose fresh, raw, organic, whole foods that contain EFAs and some that contain monounsaturated fats as well. Examples of such foods include:

   - All seeds and nuts that contain omega-6s (most of them), and especially higher quantities of the few that contain omega-3s. The seeds and nuts richest in omega-3s are flax, chia, hemp, and walnuts. High-fat, cold-water fish such as sardines, salmon, trout, herring, and mackerel (omega-3 derivatives)

   - Soybeans, garbanzos, lentils, and beans also contain some omega-3

   - Avocados, coconuts, and olives

   - Blue-green algae, chlorella, sprouts, leafy greens, and grass contain tiny amounts of good fats (0.1 percent)

4. Pay special attention to getting more omega-3 fats into your diet (via food or oil) than omega-6s, since the majority of the population does not eat enough omega-3s for optimal health. (Yes, that probably includes you!)

5. Incorporate carefully made oils into your diet. Look for oils that have been pressed from organically grown seeds or nuts; protected from light, air, and heat during manufacturing; packaged in dark glass bottles (dark glass allows the least amount of light through, thus protecting the oil from exposure to light; also, glass is inert and doesn't leach chemicals into the oil); boxed (again, to block out light); and refrigerated during storage at the factory, in stores, and in the home. Some undamaged healthy oils, and their EFA contents, are:

- Flaxseed oil: lots of omega-3s, slightly too low in omega-6s

- Hemp seed oil: three times more omega-6s than omega-3s

- Unrefined sunflower or sesame oil: rich in omega-6s, no omega-3s

- Olive oil: lots of monounsaturated fat, no omega-3s, and low in omega-6s; look for a cold-pressed, extra-virgin olive oil

- Coconut oil: mostly saturated, and low in omega-3s and omega-6s

Good oils can be easily added to smoothies, yogurt, homemade dressings, and dips, or to cooked foods such as soups or steamed vegetables—really anything, as long as it has been removed from the heat source.

And sorry, there is no such thing as an oil that is suitable for frying. Stick with steaming, poaching, boiling, or pressure-cooking your foods, or—even better—eat them raw!

Good fats are easy to include in your diet. My go-to is Udo's Oil (a blend of flax, sesame, sunflower, and coconut oils with a ratio of 2:1 omega-3 to omega-6 fatty acids), and of course it's right in line with my raw food lifestyle. I love making my own salad dressings with Udo's Oil and sea salt!

Carol's Tip

A good fat can become a bad fat if heat, light, or oxygen damages it. Make sure to look for oils in the refrigerated section of your local natural food store, packaged in glass with a box around it (to protect it from light). And always remember to use fresh oils within two months of opening.

Is Sugar a Sweet Friend or a Nefarious Enemy?

Sugar—and high-fructose corn syrup in particular—now represents by far the largest source of calories for Americans and is a major factor in our obesity epidemic. The sugar in our food, often hidden away where you might not expect to find it, is wreaking havoc on our health.

Just take a look at the sugar consumption trends of the past three hundred years:

- In 1700, the average person consumed about 4 pounds of sugar per year.

- In 1800, the average person consumed about 18 pounds of sugar per year.

- In 1900, individual consumption had risen to 90 pounds of sugar per year.

- In 2014, more than half of all Americans consumed over half a pound of sugar per day—translating to a mind-blowing 190 pounds of sugar per year!

I had J. J. Virgin, author of *The Sugar Impact Diet,* on my show, and she explained to me that sugar is hidden in foods you would never even think of: beverages including soft drinks, fruit juices, sports drinks, and most processed foods—from packaged meats to pasta; from sauces, dips, and spreads to pretzels.

No wonder there is an obesity problem in America! According to the latest figures from the Centers for Disease Control and Prevention, 29 million Americans suffer from diabetes while another 86 million (that's a third of the population) are on a slippery slope toward becoming diabetic, called "prediabetic."

Dr. Robert Lustig, an endocrinologist from California who gained national attention after a lecture he gave titled "Sugar: The Bitter Truth" went viral in 2009, has investigated the connection between sugar consumption and the poor health of Americans and found startling results. I highly recommend watching his lecture—you can find it online—if you want to learn how sugar, especially fructose, is ruining your health biochemically.

For now, I am going to give you the basics so you know what to look out for as you read food labels, and what to buy if you have a sweet tooth or craving that you just can't ignore.

- Dextrose, fructose, and glucose are all monosaccharides, known as simple sugars. Table sugar and high-fructose corn syrup use these simple sugars in combination to create disaccharides. These are the most harmful sugars, wreaking havoc on your metabolic system and expanding your waistline. Try to avoid them.

- Sugar alcohols like xylitol, glycerol, sorbitol, maltitol, mannitol, and erythritol are neither sugars nor alcohols but are becoming increasingly popular as sweeteners. They are incompletely absorbed in your small intestine, for the most part, so they provide fewer calories than sugar but often cause problems with bloating, diarrhea, and flatulence.

- Sucralose (sold in the United States as Splenda) is not a sugar, despite its sugarlike name and deceptive marketing slogan, "made from sugar." It's a chlorinated artificial sweetener in line with aspartame (Equal, NutraSweet) and saccharin, with the detrimental health effects to match. In my opinion, these sweeteners are about the most deadly consumable substances on earth and should be avoided at all costs.

- Agave syrup was all the rage a few years ago because it supposedly has a low glycemic index and won't cause blood sugar spikes, but it is typically highly processed and contains up to 80 percent fructose—high-fructose corn syrup has less fructose than agave syrup! The end product does not even remotely resemble the original agave plant's nectar.

- Honey is about 53 percent fructose; in its processed form it is essentially the same as sugar, maybe even a little worse. But its raw form, a product easily found in health-food stores and at farmers' markets, actually has many health benefits, including antioxidants. Use it in moderation.

- Coconut sugar, brown rice syrup, and yacon root powder and syrup are all healthier alternatives to other sugars. Also, Dr. Perlmuttter recommends stevia, which is derived from a South American plant and is completely healthy in its natural state.

Whew! All that talk about sugar has made me thirsty. Let's dive right into the subject of water.

Alkaline Water

Water makes up about 75 percent of our bodies, including our brains and bones. It transports nutrients, removes toxins, and regulates body temperature. Every part of our system relies on water.

Water's benefits cannot be overstated! Simply drinking more water can boost your metabolism; keep your skin soft and supple; and help reduce the number of headaches you experience. But what if I told you the water you drink could also help your body absorb more nutrients and even help prevent illness and disease? Enter: alkaline water!

Dr. Theodore A. Baroody, author of one of my favorite health books, *Alkalize or Die,* advocates drinking alkaline water for overall better health. But what is it and how is it different from other water?

Let's begin with a quick chemistry lesson. Remember the good ole pH scale from eighth-grade chemistry class? Well, it's used to define degrees of alkalinity and acidity on a scale of 0 to 14, where a pH of less than 7 is acid, 7 is neutral, and higher than 7 is alkaline.

The body continually strives to balance its pH level—ideally we want to be between 7 and 7.35. In this range, your blood is considered to be in homeostasis, which is the ideal point of balance that allows everything to function correctly. Only when our pH is balanced can the body assimilate minerals and nutrients properly. Dr. Baroody believes that acidity in the body is at the root of many ailments: "Virtually all degenerative diseases including cancer, heart disease, arthritis, osteoporosis, kidney and gall stones, and tooth decay are associated with excess acidity in the body." Unfortunately, the standard American diet, or S.A.D., is very high in acid. Meats, dairy, processed grains, and sugar are all acidic foods, and eating too many of them turns your blood acidic. Most people's diets are 80 percent acidic and 20 percent alkaline—this should be reversed, because an acidic environment allows viruses to thrive and grow. This is where alkaline water can be helpful.

Although water is usually in the middle, and by law it has to have a pH near 7 (or neutral), you never know what's coming out of your tap, or what's in your water bottle, unless you investigate. I had Christopher Dobrowolski, owner of Live Live & Organic in New York City, on my show and we tested the alkalinity of a popular U.S. brand of bottled water. When we tested it, the pH strip was yellow (around a 5, which is a hundred times more acidic than tap water and ten thousand times more acidic than good alkaline water), meaning the water was actually very acidic. I was so surprised to see that I couldn't even rely on bottled water to be pH neutral! I realized that we must take another step to fight acidity in the body with water.

Carol's Tip

Feeling the onset of heartburn or is your heartburn getting worse while drinking alkaline water? Switch back to filtered water of a neutral pH for a week. Sometimes the body is just alkaline enough.

HOW DO I GET ALKALINE WATER?

There are several ways you can make your water alkaline. The easiest and most cost-effective way to treat your water is to purchase alkaline drops. These drops work by simply adding more alkaline mineral hydroxides to your water. Many people prefer this method because you can carry the bottle of drops anywhere—a convenient perk for me and anyone else on the go.

A second way to fight acidity is to get an alkaline water filter, also known as an ionizer. I have one in both my kitchen and bathroom! I sat down with Barbara Wilk, founder and CEO of The Water Doctor, so she could explain how her alkaline ionizer machine works:

"The device is connected directly to your faucet, either on top or under the countertop, and uses a two-step process. The first task is to filter out harmful components of the water: chlorine, trihalomethanes, phenols, sediment, odor, taste, organic waste, and bacteria of all kinds. The second task is a process of electrolysis, where the water is separated into two streams—one alkaline for drinking and the other acidic. The alkaline ionized water is for drinking and cooking. The acidic water produced by ionization is not to be consumed, but is perfect for topical applications, such as skin washing, cooking utensil cleansing, and sterilizing household surfaces—thus reducing bacteria and microbe infections."

I personally use both the alkaline drops and ionized filter to drink alkaline water. I keep my drops in my bag for when I leave my apartment and have my ionized water faucets at home for everyday use.

Another great book on this topic is *Reverse Aging,* by Sang Whang. Whang recommends drinking five glasses of alkaline water a day for three months straight. Whang's advice is what started me on my own alkaline adventure.

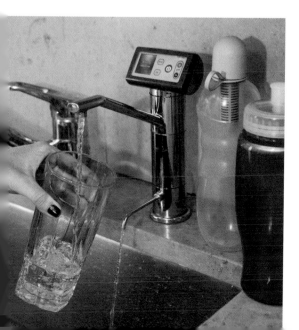

I thought drinking alkaline water would be interesting and promising, and actually a pretty easy thing to do, so I decided to try it out myself. I had been trying to alkalize my body for twenty years and this seemed like a good solution. I first checked with my doctor, Nicholas Gonzalez, MD, as anyone should before embarking on a new diet, exercise, or health plan.

After I got the go-ahead, I started drinking five glasses of alkaline water every day for three months.

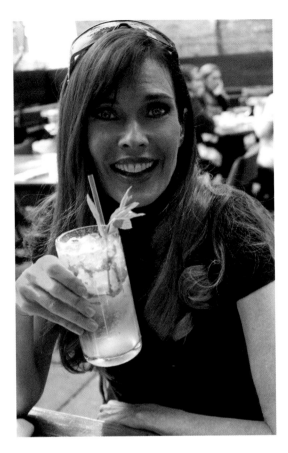

And it worked! The last time I went for blood testing, Dr. Gonzalez told me I was now too alkaline—so I would have to adjust by cutting back a little. Crazy! After two decades of trying hard to find balance, I had found a solution that worked for me, and it was as simple as adding drops to my water and using an ionizing filter.

Everyone's body is different and it is important to be monitored by a doctor along the way if you decide to try alkaline water yourself. You'll be able to work together to come up with the right pH balance for you. I promise, alkaline water could be the answer you've been waiting for.

Carol's Tip

To test your body's pH at home, purchase pH papers online. For best results, test both your saliva and urine multiple times a day (morning, afternoon, and evening, but not close to meals) for a week and bring the results to your doctor. Your pH changes all the time, but testing for a full week should give you a general idea!

Ask Carol

I've heard so many things about drinking water!
Do you have any tips you follow?

ANSWER:

- I recommend not drinking water immediately before *or* after you've eaten, because water, especially alkaline water, will dilute the enzymes in your stomach and not allow you to digest food properly.

- Drink lemon water every morning. Lemons, which taste acidic because they contain citric acid, actually have an alkalizing effect on the body.

- I purchase alkaline drops from Live Live & Organic in New York City or online at Alkalife (https://alkalifestore.myshopify.com).

- For an entire water system (best option!), I recommend contacting Jim Artress at Custom Air & Water Specialties (www.customairandwater.com) or Barbara Wilk at The Water Doctor (www.thewaterdoctor.com).

Cancer-Fighting Foods

As we just learned with alkaline water, it is important for our bodies to have a balanced pH. Cancer and most other diseases will thrive in an acidic environment in your body. An acidic environment also causes aging. If you can balance the pH of your internal body environment, you can help prevent or fend off most diseases and create a healthy climate for all of your cells.

All food can be classified as acidic or alkaline at two key stages. The first is *before* you eat it; for example, that lemon sitting on your counter is acidic. The second is how it affects your body *after* you eat it. That same acidic lemon, once it enters your body, becomes alkaline-forming. Milk, on the contrary, is naturally alkaline, but it's actually highly acid-forming in your body after you consume it.

Lemon = body alkaline = good
Milk = body acidic = bad

Confused? Well, what matters most is what the food does when it is in your body, so let's focus on that!

If your diet consists of mostly animal products and cooked and processed foods, then your internal pH is likely to be acidic, as these are all acid-forming foods. Your body is constantly trying to maintain a normal pH balance as part of homeostasis, and one of the ways it does this is by leaching calcium from your bones and teeth to neutralize high acidity. People drink processed milk for protein and calcium to build strong bones, but as we discussed, milk is acid-forming. So the body ends up taking calcium from bones and teeth to balance out the acidity caused by milk. Kinda screwy, right? The whole "milk builds strong bones" seems to me to be the opposite of what happens.

Acid-forming foods: All animal products (meats, eggs, dairy), grains, cooked food, processed foods, sugars, saturated fats, alcohol, and refined flour products like bread and pasta, and of course candy and junk food.

Alkaline-forming foods: Most raw, organic produce. I'm talking about fruits, vegetables, seeds, and nuts, as well as some beans and legumes (notice how much of the raw diet is in this list!). But remember that cooking veggies kills enzymes, destroys some nutrients, and increases acidity.

Alkaline superfoods: Tangerines, pineapple, raspberries, watermelon, limes, lentils, sweet potatoes, chlorophyll-rich dark green veggies (broccoli and kale), green powders (made up of wheatgrass, barley grass, and chlorella), apple cider vinegar, garlic, and sea salt.

Although the majority (about 95 percent) of Americans are considered acidic, there are a handful who are actually too alkaline, so it is always important to consult a doctor and check your pH level before you start anything. It's all about balance. Once you know where you

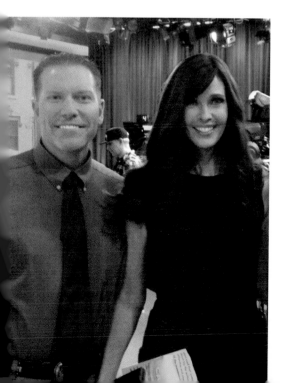

fall on the alkaline/acid scale, you can begin to adjust your eating and drinking plan to achieve your ideal pH! Don't be afraid to ask your doctor to help you start your own journey.

I asked Ty Bollinger, author of *Cancer: Step Outside the Box,* to share some of his thoughts on cancer and cancer prevention. Ty has flown all over the country talking to doctors who treat cancer and patients undergoing different procedures.

Cancer—There Is *Hope*

By Ty Bollinger

Across the globe, over 10 million people are diagnosed with cancer annually and almost 7 million die from it. According to the World Health Organization, global cancer rates could increase by 50 percent in the next fifteen years. According to a report entitled "Cancer Facts and Figures" by the American Cancer Society, 1 in 3 women alive today and 1 in 2 men alive today will face a cancer diagnosis. That's truly staggering if you think about it! The latest statistics show that one American dies of cancer every minute. That's over 1,400 people a day.

If you're like me and you've seen family members or friends suffer through conventional cancer treatments, then you know the pain and suffering they experience until the very end. Finding out that you or a loved one has cancer can be absolutely terrifying. When my father died in 1996, it inspired me to get to the bottom of what causes cancer and what treatments actually work to stop this terrible disease.

Consider these facts:

- Each year, we spray over a billion pounds of pesticides on our crops.

- We feed millions of pounds of antibiotics to our farm animals.

- We inject our cattle and livestock with cycle after cycle of growth hormones.

- We eat hundreds of pounds of genetically modified foods annually.

- We eat grains contaminated with mycotoxins (fungal toxins).

- We dump billions of tons of toxic chemicals into our waste sites and rivers.

- We drink diet sodas contaminated with aspartame.

- We have mouths full of mercury fillings and get root canals.

- We let doctors destroy our bodies with X-rays.

- We smoke cigarettes and drink lots of alcohol.

- We eat mainly junk food, fast food, and processed food.

Is it any wonder we are sick all the time?

What Causes Cancer?

Our bodies are made up of trillions of living cells. Each cell is unique, has its own identity, and performs a specific task. In the body, these trillions of cells have to interact and work together in order to maintain health and vigor. Cancer cells are constantly being created in the body, but the immune system has the ability to seek out and destroy these cells. However, tumors begin when more cancerous cells are being created than an overworked, depleted immune system can destroy. Cutting out the tumor does not usually fix the problem. Remember, a tumor is just an uncontrolled growth of cells, and is just a symptom of cancer, not the cause.

However, tumors do have the ability to migrate to different parts of the body and grow out of control there as well, so I am not saying that tumors are irrelevant. They may compress surrounding structures, and their waste products may be toxic to the rest of the body. This being so, they often interfere with the function of organs such as the brain, liver, kidney, and lungs, resulting in death. Overcoming cancer is a process of reversing the conditions that allowed the cancer to develop. In my opinion, cancer is a systemic imbalance. In other words, it is a problem with the entire system of the interrelated parts of the body. As such, appropriate treatment must be for the total environment of the body.

Why Do Some People Get Cancer and Others Don't?

Given the same exposure to the same toxins over the same period of time, someone with a healthy immune system may have no adverse effects, while someone with a compromised immune system may develop cancer. We see the evidence of this truth constantly around us. One person in an office gets a very bad cold. The one sitting next to him doesn't even get a sniffle. Certainly both were exposed to the same microorganisms. But what is the difference? One of them has a healthy immune system while the other does not.

Some people are better able to resist cellular mutations and damage by outside toxins and carcinogens. Perhaps their acid-buffering systems are better suited to maintaining homeostasis within the body's pH system. So, in spite of years of exposure to external toxins, chemicals, tobacco, and the steady consumption of a poor diet, they will not develop cancer, while others exposed to the same toxins will. Human cancer is primarily attributable to chemical pollutants, horrible eating habits, and unhealthy lifestyles.

No matter what your genetic predisposition, there are a multitude of steps you can take to minimize your cancer risk if you don't have cancer, and there are scores of successful treatment protocols you can use if you do have cancer. Knowledge is power!

Prevention Is the Key

In addition to treatments, there are also many things you can do to lower your risk for cancer. Please don't wait until you get the diagnosis—there are many preventative steps you can take now, including the following:

- Eliminate genetically modified organisms (GMOs) from your diet; they are typically treated with herbicides such as glyphosate (brand name Roundup) that are likely to be carcinogenic.

- Eat primarily raw, organic foods.

- Eliminate sugar and high-fructose corn syrup.

- Eliminate sugary beverages.

- Eliminate artificial sweeteners (like aspartame).

- Eat healthy, and preferably raw, oils (coconut oil, extra-virgin olive oil, flax oil, avocado oil, and krill oil).

- Eliminate unhealthy oils (hydrogenated oils, processed canola oil, cottonseed oil, soybean oil, and corn oil).

- Eat natural probiotics (fermented foods like sauerkraut, kefir, and miso) to optimize your gut flora, or at least take a probiotic or two daily!

- Eat and drink only raw organic dairy products.

- Eliminate wheat from your diet.

- Exercise—staying active lowers insulin levels and creates a low-sugar environment that discourages the growth and spread of cancer cells. Rebounding on a mini trampoline is an excellent choice because it stimulates lymphatic flow.

- Get the right amount of vitamin D; scientific evidence indicates that you can decrease your risk of cancer by more than 50 percent simply by optimizing your vitamin D levels.

- Get enough sleep and try to eliminate stress.

Know that how you treat your cancer is your choice, and prevention is the key!

Cancer Prevention

Ty has so many great tips on cancer prevention, but, as I mentioned, I love getting opinions from many doctors and then making my own choices about my health. I want to share some of the thoughts of premier breast cancer specialist Dr. Christine Horner, author of *Waking the Warrior Goddess: Dr. Christine Horner's Program to Protect Against and Fight Breast Cancer,* who was also a guest on *A Healthy You & Carol Alt*. She shocked the audience by sharing her view that breast cancer is a largely preventable disease. In fact, nearly 95 percent of cases can be prevented, she argues, through diet and lifestyle changes alone.

On the show, Dr. Horner emphasized the importance of prevention as a breast cancer (and cancer in general) treatment. She also shared twenty inspiring tips to lower your risk of breast cancer (which can also be applied to all cancers).

There are certain foods, nutritional supplements, and lifestyle approaches that stand out in their ability to lower your risk of cancer. Here are some of the most effective:

TIP #1:
EAT FRESH, ORGANICALLY GROWN FRUITS AND VEGETABLES—ESPECIALLY CRUCIFEROUS VEGETABLES—EVERY DAY.

Organically grown plants (especially those in the cruciferous family, for example, broccoli, cauliflower, cabbage, and kale) are filled with a variety of nutrients, vitamins, and plant chemicals that act as powerful natural medicines against breast cancer.

TIP #2:

NIX RED MEAT.

Women who eat the most red meat—especially when cooked at high temperatures or grilled—have up to a 400 percent higher risk of developing breast cancer.

TIP #3:

AVOID ALL HEALTH-DESTROYING FATS. CONSUME HEALTH-PROMOTING FATS EVERY DAY.

Saturated animal fats, trans fats, partially hydrogenated fats, and hydrogenated fats fuel breast cancer. Healthy fats—especially omega-3 fatty acids—offer protection. Supplemental flaxseed oil or purified fish oils are crucial for good health.

TIP #4:

EAT 2 TO 3 TABLESPOONS OF GROUND ORGANIC FLAXSEEDS EVERY DAY.

Flaxseeds are one of the richest plant sources of omega-3 fatty acids, are high in fiber, and contain one hundred times more cancer-fighting lignans than any other known edible plant. Supplements containing lignans are also available, such as Brevail, made by Barlean's.

TIP #5:

DRINK GREEN TEA EVERY DAY OR TAKE IT AS A SUPPLEMENT.

Women who drink green tea have a much lower risk of breast cancer—and if they get breast cancer, their chances of surviving are much greater.

Carol's Tip

Make sure your green tea is organic! Some producers use propyl glycine or formaldehyde to process their teas. Thanks to Zhena from Gypsy Tea for that information!

TIP #6:
CONSUME TURMERIC EVERY DAY.

Almost 7,000 studies have documented turmeric's potent anticancer properties, which include powerful anti-inflammatories and antioxidants. Inhibiting the growth of over seventeen different kinds of cancer, turmeric is considered "the number one anticancer spice" by Dr. Horner.

TIP #7:
TAKE AN IMMUNE-BOOSTING MEDICINAL MUSHROOM SUPPLEMENT CALLED AHCC.

Active hexose correlated compound (AHCC) has been the subject of hundreds of studies showing that it supports every cell type in the immune system and lowers the risk of numerous types of cancer, including breast cancer. AHCC is prescribed in hospitals in Japan because it significantly improves survival and takes away many of the side effects of chemotherapy.

TIP #8:
INCLUDE SEAWEED IN YOUR DIET.

Wakame and mekabu seaweeds are high in the mineral iodine, which research shows is more effective at killing breast cancer cells than many common chemotherapeutic drugs.

TIP #9:
TAKE A VITAMIN SUPPLEMENT EVERY DAY.

Certain vitamins—especially vitamin B$_{12}$, folate, vitamin D, and vitamin E—help to prevent the growth of breast cancer. Choose a vitamin made from whole foods rather than one that is made synthetically.

TIP #10:
GET ADEQUATE AMOUNTS OF SELENIUM EVERY DAY.

As little as 200 micrograms a day of this antioxidant lowers your risk of breast cancer—and many other types of cancer—by 50 percent. Brazil nuts are an excellent source. You can also take selenium as a supplement.

TIP #11:
AVOID REFINED SUGAR—USE A NATURAL SWEETENER SUCH AS STEVIA INSTEAD.

Sugar is cancer's favorite food. According to Dr. Horner, the more of it you eat, the faster cancer will grow.

TIP #12:
KEEP YOUR BODY FAT LOW.

Fat cells manufacture estrogen, notably after menopause. That's why obesity is a significant risk factor for breast cancer and is thought to contribute to more than 40 percent of all postmenopausal breast cancers.

TIP #13:
RARELY, IF EVER, DRINK ALCOHOL.

Even half a glass of alcohol a day increases your risk of breast cancer, so it's best to avoid this dangerous beverage completely. Folic acid supplements diminish many of the ill effects, so if you have a glass of wine now and again, take 200 to 400 micrograms of folic acid on the days you drink.

TIP #14:
NEVER SMOKE TOBACCO PRODUCTS.

Research shows that women who smoke *or* inhale *passive* smoke have as much as a 60 to 90 percent increased risk of breast cancer.

TIP #15:
KEEP YOUR HOME AS TOXIN-FREE AS POSSIBLE.

Toxins are everywhere—in your water, clothing, furnishings, construction materials, dry cleaning, personal care products, lawn and garden products, insect repellent, flea collars, paints, wallpaper, carpeting, and tile. Assume that everything is toxic unless it is labeled otherwise and choose a nontoxic solution instead.

TIP #16:
TAKE A WEEK OR TWO, ONCE OR TWICE A YEAR, TO PURIFY YOUR BODY.

Detoxing works! Just one five-day series of the Ayurvedic purification procedures known as *panchakarma* has been shown to cut your load of toxins in half. There are also home detox programs that are effective. Eat a diet of pure organic fresh vegetables and fruits, drink plenty of purified water, and add a few detoxifying herbs such as milk thistle, turmeric, cilantro, and spirulina. Infrared saunas help boost the release of toxins.

TIP #17:
GO TO BED BY 10:00 P.M. AND GET UP BEFORE 6:00 A.M.

Melatonin, the sleep hormone, is a powerful antioxidant that arrests and deters breast cancer in many ways. Staying up past 10 p.m. significantly decreases melatonin and increases your risk of numerous diseases, including breast cancer, heart disease, diabetes, and obesity. Waking up before 6 a.m. helps you stay in tune with your body's natural clock.

TIP #18:
MINIMIZE YOUR EXPOSURE TO ELECTROMAGNETIC FIELDS (EMFS).

All electrical appliances and wires produce breast cancer–promoting EMFs. By standing just a few feet away from appliances and wires, you can avoid the EMFs' damaging effects. For electrical devices that require you to be close to them, such as hair dryers, computers, and cell phones, there are ways to minimize the harm. Hair dryers produce more EMFs than any other household appliance, so use a low-EMF dryer, such as the CHI dryer, instead.

Carol's Tip

I love my barefoot grounding pad. I sleep on one and I tuck one under my desk as well. I found that the pad creates a pathway for the EMFs to go through and out of my body—not into it and stuck!

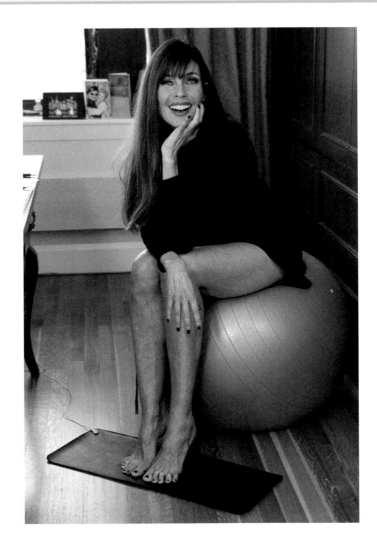

TIP #19:
EMBRACE AT LEAST THIRTY MINUTES OF AEROBIC ACTIVITY EVERY DAY.

Just thirty minutes of aerobic activity three to five times a week can lower your risk of breast cancer by 30 to 50 percent. Regular rigorous exercise can lower your risk by as much as 80 percent!

TIP #20:
PRACTICE A STRESS-REDUCING TECHNIQUE EVERY DAY.

Stress has been found to contribute to about 90 percent of all illnesses, including cancer. Research shows that the daily practice of a type of meditation called Transcendental Meditation (TM) can lower your risk of most diseases by as much as 50 percent. Tai chi, qigong, and yoga are great stress-busters, too. The regular practice of special breathing exercises called *pranayama* improves stress-hormone balance, blood pressure, heart rate, and cholesterol levels.

According to Dr. Horner, if you adopt just one of these health habits, you can cut your breast cancer risk by 50 percent! When you add another, the protective effects don't just add together, they multiply. So, it becomes incredibly simple to dramatically lower your breast cancer risk. It's a remarkable thing to realize the power you have over your own health.

Probiotics are organisms such as bacteria or yeast that are believed to improve health. I asked Dr. Udo Erasmus to share some quick facts on why probiotics are so important!

Probiotics

By Udo Erasmus, PhD

Why Are Probiotics Supplements Helpful?

1. They produce molecules in the gut that improve immune function.

2. They stimulate gut cells to make a slippery, protective mucin layer for the inner lining of the digestive tract.

3. They fight bad bacteria (*E. coli,* salmonella, and others) by stealing their food, inhibiting their growth, outpopulating them, and preventing them from making toxins that tax the immune system.

4. They lower blood pressure, blood sugar, cholesterol, and cortisol by reducing damage within the digestive tract.

5. And they help people with stress-related disorders such as depression and anxiety, IBS, and neurodevelopmental disorders such as autism via the microbiome-brain-gut axis, according to recent research.

How Do I Choose the Most Effective Probiotics?

1. Emphasize human-source probiotics. Nature adapted these to be most at home in our gut, and to withstand strong human stomach acids and bile. They implant in our gut walls, living and reproducing there for an average of about two weeks.

2. Dairy probiotics, such as those in yogurt, are useful but transient (they don't implant). Because they're designed for a calf's less acidic lower bile digestive system, up to 90 percent or more of dairy probiotics are destroyed by human stomach acids and bile (even still, dead probiotics have some benefits).

3. Buy only refrigerated probiotics. True probiotics do not form spores that survive for a long time, so they need the extra protection of low temperatures.

4. Buy blends. Like humans, probiotics work better in teams than alone.

5. Buy condition-specific blends. Different conditions respond to different blends. For travelers: Lactobacilli most effectively fight bad foreign bacteria. For lower bowel problems: Bifidobacteria most effectively protect the colon.

How Do I Best Use Probiotics?

1. Mix probiotics into foods that are not too hot to eat. In nature, probiotics found on fresh, raw foods start to work in the mouth, and continue their work throughout the entire digestive tract. The higher up they start, the more benefits you get. Most people swallow capsules, and then miss some benefits.

2. Keep probiotics refrigerated. If you travel without refrigeration, know that you'll lose about 2 percent of your supply per day.

3. Take probiotics before, during, and after antibiotic treatments to prevent reinfection by unfriendly bacteria.

Juicing and Blending

I'm constantly being asked which is better for your health, juicing or blending? The short answer: both! I personally like juicing more than blending, since it does more to make the body alkaline. The body doesn't have to digest nutrients from juice; it just absorbs them, which is less stressful and less acidic for the body.

I turned to Joe Cross, aka Joe the Juicer, who starred in the successful documentary *Fat, Sick & Nearly Dead,* and Tess Masters, author of the popular book *The Blender Girl,* for some more in-depth answers.

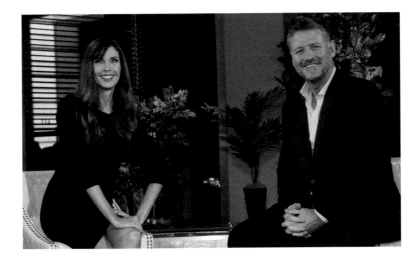

JUICING

Joe Cross knew he needed a change, which is why he set out on a sixty-day juice fast while traveling around the United States. He was *fat*— 300 pounds with a size 44 waist—and sick, suffering from an autoimmune disease that no doctor could trace back to a root cause. The disease was causing him to swell up and break out in hives on any part of his body that was subjected to pressure. This disease left him unable to do even normal everyday actions like lying down or carrying groceries.

Then juicing changed his life.

Juicing removes the insoluble fiber from vegetables and fruits. While fiber is an established, important part of an overall healthy diet, removing the insoluble fiber allows for increased absorption of specific health-promoting phytonutrients including enzymes. Meanwhile, the soluble fiber remains in the juice. Consuming fruits and vegetables in liquid form provides a nutrient delivery system for individuals who might otherwise have difficulty consuming whole fruits and vegetables and miss the opportunity to reap the numerous benefits they have to offer.

Joe explains, "Juicing offers many life-enhancing health benefits, including a faster, more efficient way to absorb immune-boosting nutrients naturally found in fruits and vegetables. It provides a way to access digestive enzymes typically locked away in the fiber matrix of whole fruits and vegetables. Most commercial juices are processed and lacking in nutrition, while freshly juiced fruits and vegetables are loaded with an abundance of vitamins, minerals, and phytonutrients."

Joe kindly shared this amazing recipe with me!

JOE'S MEAN GREEN JUICE

Makes one 16-ounce serving

1 cucumber

4 celery stalks

2 apples

6 to 8 leaves kale

½ lemon

1 tablespoon fresh ginger

1. Wash all produce well.

2. Peel the lemon (optional).

3. Put all the ingredients into a juicer and juice.

4. Pour the juice into a glass filled with ice and serve.

Joe recommends making fresh juice a part of a well-balanced, plant-based diet. It is clearly an important tool for achieving good health.

For people too sick to fully digest food, juicing is one way to try to bring them back to health.

BLENDING

On the other hand, Tess Masters admits to both juicing and blending on a regular basis. She believes they are both an important part of a healthy diet. Tess was diagnosed with the Epstein-Barr virus as a teenager, which changed the way she viewed food. Her doctor recommended she give up wheat and dairy, and when she complied, she saw a dramatic improvement in her life. After trying out all kinds of diets over twenty years, she realized there is no "one size fits all" approach and developed her own "Tess diet," which incorporated a lot of blending. In 2010, she started a successful blog and became known as the "Blender Girl."

Tess doesn't just blend smoothies; she blends full meals, snacks, appetizers, and even household cleaners. I encourage you to check out Tess's blog at www.healthyblenderrecipes.com for helpful tips and recipes. One of my favorites is her Tastes-Like-Ice-Cream Kale Shake.

TASTES-LIKE-ICE-CREAM KALE SHAKE

Makes two 16-ounce servings

½ cup filtered water

½ cup raw unsalted cashews, soaked for 2 hours, then drained

1 cup torn-up curly green kale leaves (1 or 2 large leaves with stalk removed, torn into small pieces)

2 ripe bananas

¼ cup chopped pitted dates

½ teaspoon minced ginger, plus more to taste

½ teaspoon natural vanilla extract

2 cups ice cubes

Throw the ingredients into your blender and blast on high for about 1 minute, or until smooth and creamy.

SO, WHAT'S THE MAIN DIFFERENCE BETWEEN THE TWO?

With blending, you're using the entire fruit or vegetable, including the skin and seeds, which means the resulting drink or smoothie is full of fiber. With juicing, you are extracting the juice, which is the water and most of the nutrients the produce contains, but leaving the fiber behind. Tess likes keeping the fiber because it helps to clean out her digestive tract and get rid of toxins. Blended smoothies still have all the nutritional benefits of juicing but also tend to be more filling because of the fiber. Juicing, however, allows for easy absorption.

Ask Carol

Do you have a go-to smoothie or juice recipe?

ANSWER:

I like to juice cucumbers, celery, and an apple.

I also make blended meals with raw powders (I use VITOS Go Shake), hemp seed powder, almond butter, a little water, and honey.

My favorite blend is from Dr. Timothy Brantley, the first doctor who taught me the power of raw food. Combine raw milk, green powder, 1 Thai (young) coconut (both the meat and water), raw butter, and honey.

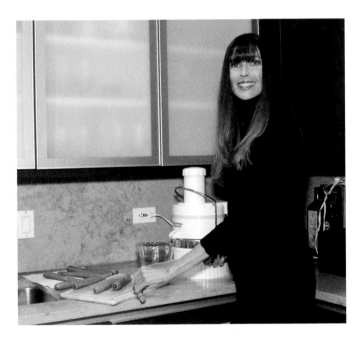

The Great Coffee Debate

Coffee: Is it good or bad for you? There is a lot of conflicting research and studies on coffee, so it's no wonder everyone is confused. It sometimes seems to be simultaneously the cause of and cure for everything.

Personally, I'm anti–drinking coffee (as you read on you'll see what I mean by this). I don't think it has any redeeming health qualities. As you've read in the previous sections, most people have overly acidic bodies, and acid is the cause of just about all disease, aging, and inflammation. Why would I want to drink something that is going to make me more acidic?

I know what you are thinking: "But, Carol, what about the antioxidants in coffee? Isn't it healthy for me?" My opinion is, even if coffee had four thousand times the antioxidants we need, I would not drink it because it is also just about four thousand times more acidic than is good for the body. Period. There are many other ways to get these antioxidants—especially from eating foods raw. And don't forget about the chemicals involved in processing regular coffee—and decaf coffee uses even more chemicals!

Let's turn to an expert, Dr. Nicholas Gonzalez:

> "Another problem with coffee is that it kicks your adrenals. In this day and age of high stress, which forces adrenals to work overtime, it is not good for the system to also be synthetically forced into responding. The body cycles from alkaline to acid to alkaline to acid all day long; the time between 2 and 4 p.m. is an alkaline cycle, for example. That means we feel more tired or more relaxed, not as energetic, between those hours. If we are not accepting of these cycles, we will turn to coffee to kick us into motion. Since

this goes against the body's natural cycle, coffee kicks the adrenals. It falsely stimulates them, to give you energy in a moment when we should be relaxing into an alkaline cycle. This is clearly not good for the body. Besides, since your adrenals regulate some hormones, forcing them to work can force them to kick out extra hormones. That overflow of hormones unbalances the body and can lead to disease."

The bottom line is: Be aware of how coffee affects your own body. If, for example, you drink coffee in the morning and have to run to the bathroom right away, this is probably a sign that something isn't right. Trust yourself; listen to what your body is telling you and be proactive about it.

Ask Carol

I want to quit coffee but I love the taste. Do you suggest any alternatives?

ANSWER:
Try the healthy acid- and caffeine-free alternatives like those from Teeccino, which makes herbal teas that taste similar to coffee but don't have its negative side effects.

"BUT WAIT, YOU ONLY SAID YOU DON'T *DRINK* COFFEE . . ."

You're probably still wondering what I meant by "I don't *drink* coffee." Well, if you watch my show you know that I use coffee another way—in an enema!

Yes, you read that right. Coffee enemas. They are not as scary as you think. They have actually been done at home for centuries. Coffee enemas are extra special because they detox not just the colon (as most enemas do) but also stimulate your liver. You can also do them easily in the comfort of your own home.

Your liver is your body's gatekeeper. Everything you eat, drink, and breathe is filtered there and either absorbed or eliminated. Unfortunately, many people don't treat their livers right (for example, by eating processed food and drinking alcohol), so they are overworked. Coffee enemas help kick them back into gear.

Coffee enemas were first popularized by Max Gerson, MD, author of *A Cancer Therapy: Results of Fifty Cases.* Dr. Gerson pioneered nutritional therapy for cancer and other diseases with excellent results. His therapy combined coffee enemas with a special diet, juices, and other supplements. The enemas were an integral part of the therapy. They are also utilized by Dr. Nicholas Gonzalez and Dr. Linda Isaacs, a board-certified internist, in their practices today.

I spoke with Dr. Isaacs about the effects of coffee enemas, and she said: "Coffee enemas have a positive effect on the whole gastrointestinal tract." They help reduce levels of toxicity in your body, relieve constipation and insomnia, increase energy levels, fight sluggishness and cognitive problems; they also eliminate (or control) parasites, candida, and other pathogens without disrupting intestinal flora.

How It Works

Dr. Isaacs explained how coffee enemas work: "The coffee enters the colon and is absorbed by the veins that are the closest to the liver. The caffeine in the coffee stimulates the liver and gallbladder to contract. The purpose of that contraction is to force out old bile. Your body is brilliant and it reutilizes bile over and over again. This old bile, when we reutilize it, may have bacteria in it and residual toxins. By forcing the bile out of the liver into the intestines to be washed away, the body is forced to make new clean bile each time, which keeps the body clean."

How to Make a Coffee Enema

To perform a coffee enema at home, you will need:

2 tablespoons organic dark
   roast coffee grounds
1 quart of purified filtered
   water
1 tablespoon blackstrap
   molasses (optional)
enema kit
personal lubricant
towel

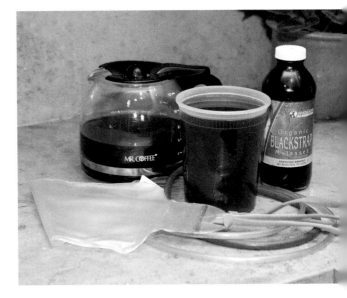

1. The night before, brew the coffee in a coffee maker using one quart of purified water with two tablespoons of caffeinated coffee grinds.

2. Add molasses to the hot coffee to thicken it if you think that you will have trouble holding the coffee for 10 minutes.

3. Let the coffee cool overnight.

4. In the morning, heat the coffee to body temperature (never hotter!).

5. Put the soft rubber tip on the enema bag and fill the bag with the coffee. Apply personal lubricant to the rubber tip.

6. Lie on your left side with the towel under your body, insert the tip, and slowly release half the bag's contents.

7. Work your way up to holding the coffee for 10 minutes.

8. Release the coffee into the toilet.

9. Repeat with the second half of the coffee.

Don't feel squeamish—the enema is eliminating waste from your body. You are just aiding your body so it can function at its best. But remember, always consult a specialist if you have any questions or anytime you are not sure if a procedure is right for you.

Grocery Shopping for Success

Time to shop now—my favorite! Are you one of those people who strolls down the supermarket aisles, adding anything to your cart no matter how good or bad it may be? Or do you get overwhelmed by all the different options and food labels?

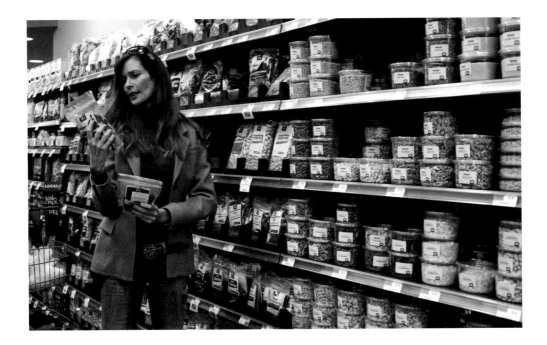

What you buy at the grocery store has a major impact on what you (and your family) eat. Health starts with smart choices. Educate yourself and be prepared next time you go grocery shopping. Trust me—it can be fun!

I recently went grocery shopping with Layne Lieberman, registered dietitian, author, and former director of nutrition for the King Kullen supermarket chain. Her number one tip? Shop the perimeter. The perimeter of a grocery store has all the fresh food—vegetables, fruits, dairy products, eggs, meat, nuts, and poultry—while less healthy, processed foods are shelved in the aisles. Sticking mostly to the perimeter will help you make the healthiest choices.

Here are some of Layne's tips for tackling food temptations and choosing healthy options:

- **Never go grocery shopping while hungry.** You will want everything and will have less willpower to resist temptation. This always ends badly, resulting in impulse purchases that otherwise would not end up in the shopping cart.

- **Plan ahead:** Choose what you are going to prepare for the week and keep a shopping list. It's a good idea to keep a running list; when you run out of something, just add it to the list. Shopping from a list keeps you focused on buying what you need and saves time and money. Make sure your list includes healthy snack options like cut-up carrots, natural nut butters, and seasonal fresh fruit.

- **Produce:** Buy local, seasonal, and organic when available. Organic foods are more regulated than conventionally produced foods, and by choosing organic you avoid pesticides, synthetic chemicals, and added hormones. There are certain produce items that you should always buy organic, such as apples, strawberries, grapes, celery, peaches, spinach, sweet bell peppers, imported nectarines, cucumbers, cherry tomatoes, imported snap peas, potatoes, hot peppers, and blueberries.

- **Bread:** If you must have bread, the secret is that breads found in the freezer aisles often have fewer preservatives and more whole-grain goodness. You are more apt to find sprouted grain, gluten-free, low-sodium, and other healthy alternatives stored in the freezer because their lack of preservatives and abundance of whole grains make these products more perishable than shelf-stable conventional varieties that are full of stabilizers and mold inhibitors. If you can't buy from a local bread baker, then this is your best option.

- **Meat:** If you can't buy organic, 100 percent grass-fed or pasture-raised meat, which is full of heart-healthy omega-3 fatty acids, buy the leanest cuts available. Fatty meats tend to hold pesticides, so choosing leaner cuts exposes you to fewer pesticides. Pigs and chickens do need some grain in their diets, so choose organic-fed and pasture-raised varieties of pork and poultry.

Carol's Tip

Bread is a tough food to give up if you've gone raw. While Ezekiel bread is cooked, it has many sprouted ingredients and can be a good alternative to processed white bread. Another option is Manna Bread (manna from heaven!), which stays raw on the inside even if the crust gets a bit cooked. Manna Bread comes in so many flavors, even some that can be used as a dessert! Try the Fruit & Nut or Cinnamon Date. The Whole Rye or Multigrain Manna Bread is great for sandwiches.

Reading Labels

Grocery stores are lined with products claiming they are good for you. Be careful of marketing! It's important to be educated about the food you are purchasing, which means being able to properly read labels. There are a lot of food trends and mislabeling of foods that make it easy to get tricked into buying something you think is healthy for you but actually isn't.

I turned to one of my favorite investigators, the author of *The Food Babe Way*, Vani Hari, to get help deciphering what different words on labels mean.

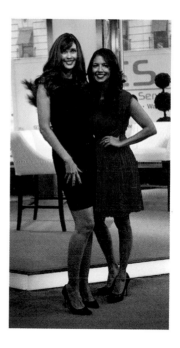

- **Low-fat, low-sugar, or low-salt:** Stay away! Just because a food product is low in one area doesn't mean it isn't loaded with other controversial ingredients. Labels such as "low-fat," "low-sugar," or "low-salt" are virtually meaningless when it comes to explaining a food's nutritional value. For example, the creators of "Reduced Fat Oreos" added more sugar to these cookies in the place of the removed fat, making this "low-fat" treat potentially even more detrimental to your health and waistline.

- **No trans fats:** Even if a package advertises "no trans fats," be careful. Products carrying this label can still have up to half a gram of trans fat per serving, according to the U.S. Food and Drug Administration (FDA). If you eat more than the suggested serving (which most people do), those fats can add up. Trans fats are a type of unsaturated fat that raises your LDL cholesterol levels (the "bad" kind) and increases your risk of heart disease. According to the Centers for Disease Control and Prevention, trans fats can be linked to 7,000 deaths and 20,000 heart attacks each year.

- **Natural:** The FDA has no formal definition for what "natural" means. This means that food created in a laboratory or food that contains artificial ingredients can be labeled "natural." A litany of class-action lawsuits have been waged against products marketed as natural that contain genetically modified organisms (GMOs)—including Goldfish crackers, Naked Juice drinks, and Kashi cereal—but the FDA has not designated GMOs as "unnatural." Additionally, Kraft defended the use of the word "natural" on different varieties of its Crystal Light products that contain artificial sweeteners, artificial colors (some made from petroleum products), and synthetic ingredients. They can call their product natural because there is no enforceable law against doing so. This is why it's absolutely critical to read the full ingredient list on all products labeled "natural."

- **Organic:** The U.S. Department of Agriculture (USDA) has specific guidelines that food producers must comply with if they want to use the "organic" label. Animal products cannot be given antibiotics or growth hormones, and plants cannot be grown with conventional pesticides or fertilizers made with synthetic ingredients or sewage. For plants to be considered organic, genetic engineering and irradiation, which exposes crops to radiation to kill bacteria and other pests, are prohibited.

Understanding the Three Levels of Organic Labeling:

* "100%" means products are made entirely from organic ingredients.

* "Organic" means that at least 95 percent of a product's ingredients are organic.

* "Made with organic ingredients" indicates that at least 70 percent of the ingredients are organic.

- **Pasteurized:** Flash pasteurization uses heat to destroy harmful bacteria, viruses, molds, and other microorganisms in a food product to help safeguard our health. But during the pasteurization process, raw enzymes, minerals, and vitamins are also killed by heat. Heat kills the bad stuff *and* the good stuff, making the product less nutritious. This is why eating an abundance of raw plant foods is absolutely critical to maintaining a nutritious diet.

Carol's Tip

Watch out for "partially pasteurized" on food labels—heat is heat! Enzymes, vitamins, and minerals are still denatured.

- **Cold-pressed, expeller-pressed oils:** It is important to look for cold-pressed oils, which are extracted using little or no heat. Traditional oils like soybean, corn, and canola can be made using controversial chemicals like hexane. Expeller-pressed oils are another safe option that doesn't use hexane. Always choose certified organic oils, because they cannot be processed using any synthetic ingredients.

- **Made with whole grains or multigrain:** These are among the most misleading terms the food industry uses on cereals, crackers, cookies, and bread. A product labeled with either of these terms can contain more refined white flour than actual whole wheat flour or whole-grain flour. Again, it's important to read the ingredients label to make sure you know what's in the products you buy.

Educate yourself and know what you are putting in your grocery basket!

My Thoughts on GMOs

I hear a lot of confusion when it comes to genetically modified organisms (GMOs) in this country. Most people don't even know what they are!

According to Max Goldberg of Livingmaxwell.com, "GMOs (or genetically modified organisms) are living organisms whose genetic material has been artificially manipulated in a laboratory through genetic engineering. This relatively new science creates unstable combinations of plant, animal, bacteria, and viral genes that do not occur in nature or through traditional crossbreeding methods."

Did you know that sixty countries have significant restrictions on GMOs or have banned them altogether, including Japan and Australia? In fact, canned fruit salads containing papaya exported to Germany and sardines in soybean oil exported to Greece and the Netherlands were recently banned because of the threat of contamination by GMOs.

Yet, the United States government says GMOs are fine for us? It seems whenever anyone questions this, it all gets passed to the FDA. Guess who the head of that organization is: Michael R. Taylor, who once worked as a lobbyist for the agribusiness giant—and leader of the pack regarding GMOs—Monsanto. Monsanto is an agricultural biotechnology corporation based in the United States and the largest producer of genetically engineered (GE) seeds.

Speaking of Monsanto, its genetically modified corn and glyphosate-based herbicide, called Roundup, was studied for two years by the French scientist Gilles-Eric Seralini. He found that Roundup caused increased disease and tumor growth in rats. Seralini's subjects were the same kind of rats that most scientists use to study cancer. There is usually a 15 to 20 percent incidence of cancer when the rats are fed "regular" food; however, that percentage increased to 80 percent for rats that were fed foods containing GMOs, with most of the female rats developing breast cancer.

I often wonder why our government is so captive to nonrenewable, debt-increasing foods. There is research that organic farming produces as much food as the conventional methods (including GMOs) yield.

According to an agricultural census taken by the USDA every five years, farms today are getting larger, up to 434 acres, even though the overall number of farms is decreasing. The value of their crops and livestock is increasing. Farms sold almost $395 billion in products in 2012, up 33 percent from 2007.

And yet, farming is considered a negative economy. Why? One big reason is that seeds are no longer considered property of the farm; rather they have become a corporate (and GMO) commodity. Seeds are now patented and engineered, need pesticides and fertilizers to grow properly, and can only be used for one year. Because farmers can't save any seeds to plant the following year, they have to increase their debt by buying more seeds every year.

And another thing? GMOs use more of the pesticides, herbicides, and chemicals that are killing bees and many other insects vital for a thriving ecosystem. In my view, there should never be a risk to consider when we're talking about eating or growing food. None of this makes sense to me! At the very least, GMOs need to be labeled. We have a right as consumers to know what we are putting in our bodies. For more information check out the documentary *GMO OMG* by Jeremy Seifert.

Following proper nutrition and eating real foods are not new ideas. Back in 400 B.C., Hippocrates said, "Let food be your medicine and medicine be your food." If we have had this guiding principle for so long, why have we, as a society, strayed so far away from it? We have chosen convenience over our health. It's time to change this behavior! I believe that proper nutrition should start at an early age; we should teach and inspire our youth to know the source of the food they are eating and the value it adds to their lives.

But it's also never too late to make changes in your own life. Use the techniques you've learned in this section and take an active role in your own health. Try incorporating more raw unprocessed foods into your meals, learn what diet is best for your body, add some smoothies or juicing to your eating habits, and be careful of your alcohol and coffee consumption—moderation is key. Take the time to learn what you're spending your hard-earned money on at the grocery store. All of these small steps will add up to a healthier you.

Invest in your health through the food you put into your body! It's the most important investment you will ever make.

PART 2

Fitness

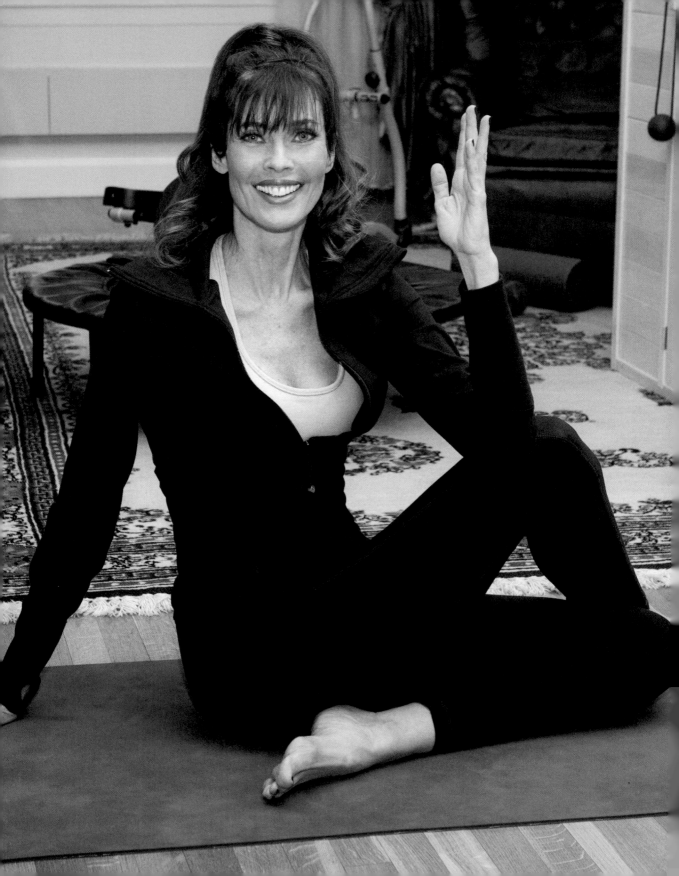

*A*fter years of interviewing top-notch health and wellness experts, reading up on cutting-edge research, and experimenting in my own life, I've discovered something pretty amazing—the basic foundation for optimal health is actually quite simple. I've realized that looking for a quick fix only complicates things!

The key to success? Eat real food (mostly vegetables), drink fresh water, and exercise daily.

But, as you probably know, when you throw your kids, a partner or spouse, a career, your family, friends, pets, and a to-do list into that simple equation, things get complicated in a hurry. Not to mention that as you get older, balancing everything seems to get more difficult!

We've been focusing on nutrition, the "what to eat" part of the equation, but now it's time to shift gears and focus on another part: fitness. We all know that fitness is important and that we should exercise regularly, but why is it so hard to motivate yourself sometimes? How can you possibly make time in your busy schedule? And are all exercises created equal? Or are there some that are more effective given inevitable time constraints? What are the benefits to my mind and body? How long should you be exercising for? How many times a week?

In this part of the book, we will explore all of these questions (and more!) with leading experts in the fitness industry. I can't wait to show you all of the exciting ways you can get your body moving! Fitness is a lifelong journey and can be a positive force in your life. By taking time to focus on your physical health, you are doing something that will benefit you, your family, and even your career. Let's find the right fitness path and learn how to make it fun, together!

Make Fitness a Priority, Not an Option

I can't tell you how many times I've heard people say "exercise starts on Monday!" Or make the infamous New Year's fitness resolution! You start out strong, maybe by joining a gym or going to a new exercise class, but eventually your initial enthusiasm and energy wane as everything else going on in your life distracts you from your goals. Soon exercising takes a backseat and you forget all about it. Why does fitness tend to be the first to-do we skip on our list as soon as we feel too busy or overwhelmed? If this is you, don't beat yourself up. Even I did it—but not anymore!

I had to retrain my mind in order to be able to stick to my exercise routine. Fitness should be a priority, not an option in our daily lives. As I've said, your health should be your number one focus, because you won't be able to do everything else you love to do—like playing with your kids, or enjoying a favorite hobby, or getting that big promotion—if you don't have your health. It's the basis for everything. Exercise is part of the equation that's going to get you there. It should be as much a part of your daily regimen as combing your hair, checking your email, or even eating. I love to work out in the morning right after I brush my teeth. It's now a part of my daily routine and I don't even thinking about *not* doing it. I actually look forward to it.

Most of us have become experts at finding reasons why we can't exercise. I used to be like that—an excuse machine! When I was modeling, my favorites were that I was too exhausted from shoots or just didn't have time in my busy schedule. (Ironically, as you will learn as you read on, exercise actually increases your energy.) On days when I finally did make it to the gym I faced another roadblock—I didn't know what to do when I got there. Should I run on a treadmill for thirty minutes? Do a hundred sit-ups? Stretch before or after riding a stationary bike? Cardio or weight lifting first? It ended up becoming too stressful to face these never-ending questions. And wouldn't you know it, the confusion just gave me another convenient excuse to stop and give up. I thought exercise just wasn't for me.

This cycle continued for years until I realized my health wasn't improving as much as it could be. Although I had the raw, healthy food part down, I was still missing the exercise part of the equation, so my overall health wasn't where it should be. I had to adjust my attitude toward working out and stop the excuses. You'll never find the right time to work out if you hate what you're doing. I set out to find a plan I enjoyed and could commit to.

I also educated myself on the amazing benefits of fitness. If you are exhausted all the time, as I was, exercise might actually be what's missing. It's hard to take that first step, but trust me—just put your shoes on or play some music! It works! Initially you might be tired, but eventually your endorphin levels will increase and you'll have more energy for the rest of the day.

In your twenties, you can get away with not exercising, because your metabolism is naturally faster. But as you get older, the same rules don't apply anymore. By the time you reach your early thirties, your metabolism starts to slow down and the differences between those who exercise and those who don't start to show, and I don't mean just in physical appearance. Of course we all want to *look* good, but exercising is about so much more. It's essential to your overall health, especially as you age! Just because you may have skated through your twenties and thirties without setting foot in a gym or exercise class doesn't mean anything once you hit middle age. Without exercise it's impossible to stay slim and healthy. I remember watching an interview with Jennifer Lopez on *E! News* where she was asked what her "secret" was to looking so good in her forties. (Again, everyone is looking for the secret quick fixes!) She hit the nail on the head by responding: "It's not easy to look good as you get older; there are no shortcuts. You have to put in the work!"

Jennifer's put in the work and it's paid off—have you seen her abs? She looks better now in her forties than she ever has!

It became so clear for me—if you don't put in the work and effort, you will not get the results you're looking for. I found my motivation by connecting the dots and learning exactly how exercise could affect my body *and* mind. When you are more conscious and aware of exercise's exact benefits, you are more likely to work out. Next time you're weighing your options, between, say, putting on your sneakers or sitting watching TV, remember that regular exercise has many physical benefits—weight control, better sleep, boosting energy levels—but it also helps fight off health issues such as heart disease, diabetes, arthritis, and cancer. Try getting those benefits from the couch!

And don't think because you are in your forties or fifties you are already too late to the exercise game and you should just give up. It's never too late to have a love affair with fitness, no matter what age you are when you start. There are so many new ways to get moving at all ages and fitness levels. Start now and don't look back!

The Many Benefits of Exercise

I've already mentioned a few amazing benefits of staying physically active, but let's really dig in to just how important staying fit is. Next time you start to think about skipping your workout, replace that list of excuses with these lists of amazing benefits.

According to the 2014 Physical Activity Guidelines for Americans, being physically active on a regular basis:

- Improves your chances of living longer and healthier

- Helps protect you from developing heart disease and stroke (not to mention their precursor, high blood pressure)

- Helps protect you from developing certain cancers, including colon and breast cancer, and lung and endometrial (uterine lining) cancer

- Helps prevent type 2 diabetes (what was once called adult-onset diabetes) and metabolic syndrome (a constellation of risk factors that increase the chances of developing heart disease and diabetes)

- Helps prevent osteoporosis

- Improves cognitive function

- Relieves symptoms of depression and anxiety and improves mood

- Prevents weight gain and promotes weight loss

- Improves heart-lung and muscle fitness

- Improves sleep

- And for me, exercise clears my head!

Yes, please! I'll take all of that. It goes on, though—not only does exercise improve your physical well-being, it also affects your mental health. Double whammy! Here are even more reasons to fight through those excuses:

The Five Mental Benefits of Exercise

1. **Reduces stress.** Rough day at work? Take a walk or head to the gym for a quick workout. Working up a sweat helps manage both physical and mental stress. Exercise also increases concentrations of norepinephrine, a chemical that moderates the brain's response to stress.

2. **Boosts happy chemicals.** Exercise releases endorphins, which create feelings of happiness and euphoria. Studies have shown that exercise significantly helps people who are clinically depressed. You can get this buzz from working out for just thirty minutes a few times a week.

3. **Improves self-confidence.** Working out helps boost your confidence and makes you feel sexier. When you feel good, you give off a certain vibrancy to the world around you. Trust me, your spouse or partner will thank you!

4. **Prevents cognitive decline.** As we age, our brains get a little hazy. While exercise and a healthy diet can't cure diseases like Alzheimer's, they can help the brain fight cognitive decline. Working out helps boost the chemicals in your brain that prevent degeneration of the hippocampus, an important part of the brain for memory and learning.

5. **Boosts brainpower.** Various scientific studies have shown that cardiovascular exercise can create new brain cells and improve overall brain performance.

Yet, despite all the positive mental and physical benefits of exercise, only about 30 percent of Americans get regular physical activity. It's important to remember, you are in control of your own health and you have the power to make a change. As with the food you eat, exercise is another area of your life that you are in charge of. It should be empowering to know that you have chosen to take control of your life and make health a priority—learn to love and respect your body and treat it right.

Carol's Tip

I exercise where and when I can—while watching TV and sometimes while I'm on hold on the phone. Even at my desk! I use any chance I have to sneak in a little something-something. I challenge myself to look for these moments to sneak in the right exercise—it's almost like a game now.

Find What You Enjoy

People are always asking me my secret or number one tip for staying physically fit. Because I've tried almost everything out there, magazine editors and television hosts always want to know the one thing

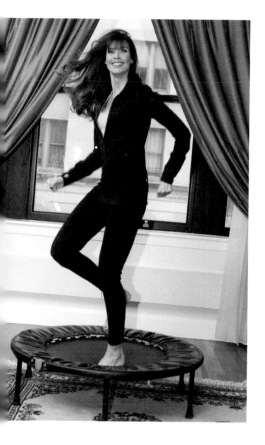

that's going to change their life when it comes to exercise. I love to answer this question because my response always shocks people.

The secret to exercise? Are you ready for it? Find an activity that you enjoy doing. It's another simple answer that we love to complicate. Exercise should be your stress release of the day, something you do for yourself, not something that stresses you out. Find an activity (or even better, a few activities) that excites you and that you look forward to every day.

It wasn't until recently that I found an exercise that I loved—yoga!

I used to dread going to the gym to work out. I hated the lighting, the people staring, the equipment I didn't know how to use and got no results from, the actual time it took to get there—it was a miserable experience start to finish. I tried to love it because I thought it was good for me, but it never stuck and just caused stress in my life. How was I supposed to make healthy exercise a priority in my life when I absolutely hated the process? I was spending too much mental energy thinking about working out, and not enough time actually doing it.

Something had to change. I was stressing over the one thing I was doing to help reduce my stress!

So I opened my mind and explored my options. When I found yoga I began to look forward to it. Imagine that! I enjoy yoga because it benefits the mind, body, and spirit. I love feeling the connection of my breath and body. It makes me feel alive and connected to the world around me. I also travel a lot, so I love that I can do it anywhere. I finally found something that works for my schedule and lifestyle and that I enjoy doing.

Exercise should not feel like a chore. You are improving your health and making your body stronger each time you put in the effort to move—whether it's walking, jogging, biking, dancing, or taking a yoga class. This simple change in mind-set can help you enjoy exercising. If you like what you're doing, I promise, it will be so much easier to find time in your busy day to do it.

Another great thing? New exercise programs are coming out every day. If you find that yoga isn't for you, you can try Pilates, Zumba, CrossFit, belly dancing, Rebounder—there's something for everyone. Even if you haven't taken a class, jogged, or gone to the gym in years, there is a program out there that can get you started.

Just to give you a sampling of what's out there to try, I talked to a few of my favorite trainers to give you a breakdown of some of the most popular exercises today.

Carol's Tip

I found that when I figured out what exercise I enjoyed, I looked forward to working out. If you find the discipline that you enjoy, maybe you will stick to it, too!

YOGA

I'm going to start with my favorite workout, yoga! To gather a little more information to inspire you to give it a go, I turned to yoga instructor Jordan Mallah to get the breakdown. Here's what I learned from Jordan.

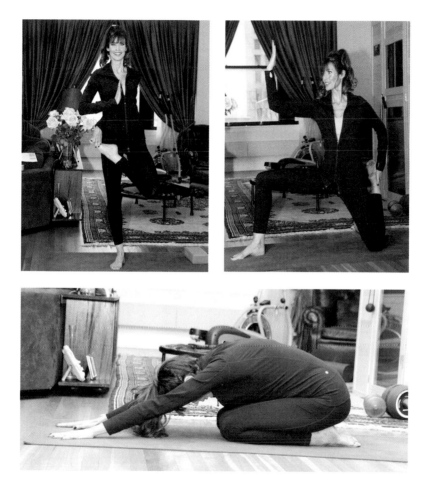

What is yoga?

Yoga is an ancient form of exercise that focuses on strength, flexibility, and breathing to boost physical and mental well-being. The word "yoga" comes from the Sanskrit word *yuj*, which means "to unite." Yoga helps you unite your mind, body, and spirit. The main components of yoga are postures—a series of movements designed to increase strength and flexibility and encourage deep breathing. The practice originated in India about five thousand years ago but has evolved in a variety of ways.

What are the health benefits of yoga?

Yoga is a safe and effective way to increase physical activity, muscle strength and tone, flexibility, and balance. There's evidence that regular yoga practice is beneficial for people with high blood pressure, heart disease, aches, pains—including lower back pain—depression, and stress. Yoga also helps improve your vitality and increases energy.

Am I too old for yoga?

Definitely not! There are yoga classes for every age group—children, teens, adults, and even seniors. The level of yoga depends on the class that you take, so be sure to do some research before you attend one.

Do I need to be flexible to do yoga?

No. Yoga is a personal practice and will help improve your flexibility to go beyond your normal range of movement no matter where you start. It is actually great for people who have tight muscles because it helps loosen them up. You'll feel more comfortable during normal daily activity.

Can I injure myself doing yoga?

The most common yoga injuries are caused by repetitive strain or overstretching. During a yoga class, it's important to start out slow and listen to what your body can handle. When you start out, make sure to go to a class where the instructor teaches you alignment and gives corrections. Learning from a qualified yoga teacher and choosing a class appropriate to your level will ensure that you remain injury-free.

What style of yoga should I do?

There are many different styles of yoga, such as Ashtanga, Vinyasa, Hatha, hot yoga, and Bikram. Some styles are more vigorous than others. Some may have a different area of emphasis, such as posture or breathing.

The key is to choose a class appropriate to your fitness level. I suggest starting out with a slow class like Hatha, which helps you learn to focus on proper alignment, and then eventually working your way up to a faster-flowing class like Vinyasa.

The following chart from *Peace Love Nutrition,* a yoga blog, can help you decide which type of yoga is best for you!

TYPE OF YOGA	PERSONALITY
Ashtanga	Ashtanga is a more vigorous style of yoga. It offers a series of poses, each held for only five breaths and punctuated by a half sun salutation to keep up the pace.
Vinyasa	Teachers lead classes that flow from one pose to the next. You usually leave with a good workout as well as a yoga experience. If you're new to yoga, it is a good idea to take a few classes in a slower style of yoga first to get a feel for the poses. Vinyasa flow is really an umbrella term for many other styles. Some studios call it flow yoga, flow-style yoga, dynamic yoga, or Vinyasa flow. It is influenced by Ashtanga yoga.
Bikram	You must love to sweat as it's in a room heated to 104°F. It's usually an hour and a half and a sequence of 26 yoga poses to stretch and strengthen the muscles as well as compress and "rinse" the organs of the body. The poses are done in a heated room to facilitate the release of toxins.
Kundalini	Kundalini yoga was designed to awaken energy in the spine. Kundalini yoga classes include meditation, breathing techniques such as alternate nostril breathing and chanting, as well as yoga postures.
Hatha	Hatha is often a gentle class. It is great for beginners as it teaches basic asanas and breathing techniques.
Yin	Yin yoga comes from the Taoist tradition and focuses on passive, seated postures that target the connective tissues in the hips, pelvis, and lower spine. Poses are held for anywhere between one and 10 minutes, The aim is to increase flexibility and encourage a feeling of release and letting go. It is a wonderful way to learn the basics of meditation and stilling the mind. As such, it is ideal for athletic types who need to release tension in overworked joints, and it is also good for those who need to relax.
Restorative	Restorative yoga is all about healing the mind and body through simple poses often held for as long as 20 minutes, with the help of props such as bolsters, pillows, and straps. It is similar to yin yoga, but with less emphasis on flexibility and more on relaxing.
Jivamukti	Founded in 1984 by David Life and Sharon Gannon, Jivamukti means "liberation while living." This is a Vinyasa-style practice with themed classes, often including chanting, music, and scripture reading. Jivamukti teachers encourage students to apply yogic philosophy to their daily life.

Carol's Tip

When I first started yoga I splurged and got a private trainer. She focused only on me, correcting my mistakes and sharing her expertise about proper form. Then I joined a class or practiced by myself at home. The personal attention at the start gave me confidence that I not only knew what a Downward-Facing Dog was, but I knew the proper form, thereby avoiding common mistakes that could cause injury. If you're venturing into your first yoga class, look for something that can offer support for beginners, and always let your instructor know if it's your first time.

Ask Carol

What is your favorite yoga mat?

ANSWER:

I love JadeYoga mats because they are made here in the United States and are made of natural rubber with no PVC. It makes me a little crazy that most people practice yoga for their health, but very few people think about what their yoga mats are made of.

Most yoga mats, even some of the most expensive ones on the market, are still made with PVC (a carcinogen) and contain phthalates (which have been banned in toys since 2008). The best way to avoid

PVC, phthalates, and other nasty chemicals when you practice yoga is to use a natural mat.

I had Dean Jerrehian from JadeYoga on my show and he recommended the four best types of mats:

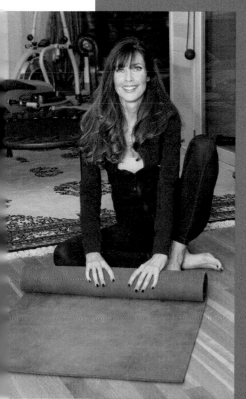

Cotton: A very soft mat made of and stuffed with cotton. This mat is very comfortable and great for meditation and floor poses. It can also be rolled up to be used as a bolster.

Rice straw: This is a beautifully woven mat that might remind you of one of those straw beach mats. Again, a great mat for meditation and floor poses.

Latex: This mat is made with latex tapped from a rubber tree. It is more like a traditional yoga mat that you might see in your yoga class. It has a nice grip and cushioning, so it would be appropriate for a wide range of yoga poses.

Rubber: This is the material JadeYoga uses for its mats. They are made with natural rubber from a rubber tree. Unlike a latex mat, a rubber mat does not have the latex proteins that cause problems for people with latex allergies.

Do you love yoga but want something more in your workouts? Check out this program from a former wrestler turned yogi!

What Is DDP YOGA?

DDP YOGA was designed by three-time World Championship Wrestler DDP, also known as Diamond Dallas Page. Dallas created a workout that feels and sounds different from traditional forms of yoga practice: DDP YOGA is a hybrid workout that combines the very best of yoga, traditional fitness, sports therapy, old-school calisthenics, and dynamic resistance while focusing on strength training, increased flexibility, and cardio. Dallas's high-energy, no-holds-barred approach to instruction resembles a boot camp workout, but these low-impact exercises can be done by anyone at any age.

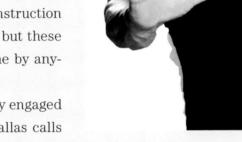

DDP YOGA poses focus on fully engaged muscular contractions, which Dallas calls "dynamic resistance." Yoga practitioners may see some familiar positions, but they are not called by their traditional Sanskrit names. Instead, Dallas has put his own twist on pose names, including his hallmark Diamond Cutter finishing move.

Just make sure you don't call it "yoga" or Dallas will get on your case—it ain't your mama's YOGA!

What Are the Health Benefits of DDP YOGA?

The main benefits of following the DDP YOGA program are body fat loss, lean muscle growth, and improved cardiovascular levels.

Dallas created DDP YOGA after a crippling injury where he ruptured his L4 and L5 discs. At age forty-two, he was told by three doctors that he would never be able to wrestle again, but the following year he won the World Championship Wrestling title! Now fifty-eight, he's in great shape, pain-free, and more flexible than ever before. Dallas says, "Flexibility is youth!"

Am I Too Old for DDP YOGA?

DDP YOGA is a workout that can be started at any age and any fitness level. But it's more than just a workout—it's a lifestyle. The more you do it, the more you'll be able to enjoy other parts of your life. If you can bend over and pick up your keys or reach up to change a lightbulb, you can do DDP YOGA!

Do I Need to Be Flexible to Do DDP YOGA?

The best part of the DDP YOGA workouts is that they allow you to modify almost any position. As long as you are engaging your muscles by using dynamic resistance, you'll still get the strength, flexibility, and cardio benefits at any exertion level. Dallas encourages people who are inflexible to try DDP YOGA. He suggests taking six "before" pictures so you can see firsthand how your body changes after thirty, sixty, and ninety days.

Can I Injure Myself Doing DDP YOGA?

Dallas created DDP YOGA to help himself recover from a back injury. These low-impact workouts can be done by anyone at any fitness level. Modify the positions as needed and make them your own!

How Do I Get Started?

Check out Diamond Dallas Page's website, http://ddpyoga.com, for more information about DDP YOGA and to order DVDs.

PILATES

If I haven't convinced you to give yoga a shot (you should!), consider trying Pilates. Pilates offers a targeted full-body workout like you've never experienced before. I reached out to Katherine and Kimberly Corp from Pilates on Fifth in New York City to help break it down. Here are some key points.

What is Pilates?

Pilates is an exercise system that focuses on stretching and strengthening the whole body to improve balance, muscle strength, flexibility, and posture. It was created by Joseph Pilates in the early 1920s and incorporates elements of yoga, martial arts, and ballet. Adopted by professional dancers in the United States as an effective form of recovery after injury, Pilates has recently grown in popularity. You can practice Pilates either on a mat or in a studio using a special apparatus.

Here's a fun fact: some of the first people treated by Joseph Pilates (to strengthen their bodies and heal their aches and pains) were dancers Martha Graham and George Balanchine.

What are the health benefits of Pilates?

Pilates can help improve posture, muscle tone and flexibility, core strength, and joint mobility, as well as relieve stress and tension.

Am I too old for Pilates?

As with yoga, you are never too old to take a Pilates class. If you can follow instructions, you can benefit from the exercises. Pilates can also be adapted to meet anyone's physical needs and goals.

"If your spine is inflexibly stiff at thirty, you are old; if it's completely flexible at sixty, you are young . . . the only real guide to your true age lies not in years, or how old you think you feel, but . . . by the degree of natural and normal flexibility enjoyed by your spine throughout life."—*Joseph Pilates*

Do I have to be fit to do Pilates?

No. Pilates is suitable for people of all levels of fitness. Practitioners say it's a more gentle way of raising your activity levels, especially if you have poor mobility, aches and pains, or an injury.

Can I injure myself doing Pilates?

Pilates is a gentle, low-impact form of exercise, and injuries are very uncommon. However, it's important that you find a qualified teacher and a class suitable to your level. If you don't exercise already or you're recovering from an injury, it's advisable to check with a health professional and the Pilates teacher before starting a class.

What's the difference between Pilates and yoga?

Both Pilates and yoga focus on developing strength, balance, flexibility, posture, and good breathing technique. With its emphasis on the unity between the mind and body, yoga has a spiritual side that Pilates does not.

Pilates uses breathing, but its exercises focus more on precise movements to target specific parts of the body and muscle groups. The best Pilates classes are in small groups where the teacher can develop programs to suit each person's strengths and weaknesses.

What's the difference between Pilates with an apparatus and Pilates on a mat?

Joseph Pilates designed his exercises to be performed on a specialized apparatus, and later developed mat exercises to allow his students to practice at home. With Pilates on mats, exercises are mostly performed on the ground, sometimes using small pieces of equipment such as stretch bands and balance balls.

Classes using the apparatus offer a higher level of individual attention from a Pilates instructor, but they're usually more expensive. The apparatus is used to provide resistance to challenge your body and support your body, depending on your needs.

TAI CHI

Want to really think outside the box to find the exercise you love? Try tai chi! If the extent of your workout is reading a magazine on a treadmill, you are in for a treat. I discussed the pros of tai chi with instructor Jonathan Angelilli. Jonathan has been teaching people movement for over fifteen years and is the founder of TrainDeep.com.

What is tai chi?

Tai chi combines deep breathing and relaxation with slow and gentle movements. Originally developed as a martial art in thirteenth-century

China, it is still practiced around the world as a health-promoting exercise. It is incredibly enjoyable and dynamic, and allows the practitioner to develop power, sensitivity, body control, and mental focus.

What are the health benefits of tai chi?

Studies have shown that tai chi can help reduce stress, improve balance and general mobility, increase muscle strength, relieve or help prevent arthritis and osteoporosis, and aid with sleep. It is even known to help you develop a more robust immune system, increase self-mastery, heighten your senses, and uncover your purpose in life.

Am I too old for tai chi?

Tai chi is commonly performed as a low-impact exercise, which means it won't put much pressure on your bones and joints and most people should be able to do it. There are more powerful variations of tai chi that are excellent for practicing fighting techniques, but the most basic (and oldest) form of tai chi, qigong, is very gentle and can be practiced by anyone at any age.

Do I need to be fit to do tai chi?

No, tai chi is for everyone who truly wants to increase mastery over their body, mind, and health. It is ideal for relatively inactive people wanting to raise their activity levels gradually because it has many benefits but is a low-impact exercise with a low risk for injury. Many of the tai chi movements can even be adapted for people with disabilities. If you can breathe and focus your mind, you can practice tai chi!

Is tai chi a form of yoga?

In a way, yes. Yoga and tai chi are like siblings. Both were developed to help practitioners improve their health, self-mastery, and ability to meditate. In general, tai chi is much gentler than yoga, and it's much harder to injure yourself while practicing basic tai chi and qigong.

Can I injure myself doing tai chi?

Tai chi is essentially a gentle activity and it's highly unlikely to cause injury if done correctly. The exercises involve lots of flowing, easy movements that don't stress the joints or muscles. Tai chi emphasizes mindful body control, and also follows the pleasure principle—if it doesn't feel good, it's not tai chi. If you listen to your body, you'll avoid injury. In fact, tai chi is excellent for improving your ability to sense and interpret your body's feelings and sensations. In the long run, this helps you avoid not only injuries but also sickness and mistakes resulting from general lack of body awareness.

Are there different styles of tai chi?

Yes, there are, such as Chen, Yang, and Wu. These are the last names of families that have passed down their unique understanding of "the way." Teachers often practice a combination of styles. Some people consider Chen to be the "original style." It was established in central China's Chen village in the seventeenth century, but the roots of tai chi are much older. Chen is the most athletic and physically difficult style, incorporating jumping kicks and stamping actions. The Yang style, which has many variations, originated from the Chen style and is the most widely practiced type of tai chi today. The Wu style, which was developed directly from the Yang, is the second most popular style. It emphasizes smaller, more compact movements than the Yang and incorporates more internal chi work.

How do I get started?

Tonight, while lying on your bed before going to sleep, put your hand on your belly and breathe deep enough—calmly and slowly—to move your hand while at the same time relaxing your mind. Lengthen your breath gently, and count each breath for five minutes. You've just started your healing tai chi practice! Of course, this is just the very beginning. The practice will teach you how to be relaxed and in control even while moving your whole body, first in simple ways and then with increasingly dynamic movements. It's a great idea to watch a class or attend a trial session before signing up for a course. Find a teacher who inspires you. It's very difficult to learn the deeper and most powerful aspects of the tai chi practice by reading books and watching videos; it's such an experiential practice based on the energy exchange between student and teacher. Heart to heart, from teacher to student—this is the way each tai chi lineage has passed down its wisdom for centuries!

ZUMBA

Do you love to dance but haven't even tried since you were young or out at a club? Working out should be fun, and you can dance your way to better health through Zumba! Bessie Neshan from Carve Your Body, in Emerson, New Jersey, shared her Zumba secrets with me. Here's what I learned.

What is Zumba?

Zumba is a worldwide fitness phenomenon. Started in 2001, Zumba is a feel-good, dance/aerobic workout that combines easy moves, motivating music, and high energy to exercise your body and mind. No dance experience is needed. Everyone follows the instructor in moves and combinations that are fun and easy.

Zumba classes appeal to both men and women of all ages, from teens to seniors, and is effective for a range of fitness levels. Over the years, Zumba has morphed into a variety of class formats to satisfy people's needs. Bessie said she feels this is one reason for Zumba's lasting popularity—it's constantly evolving. Workouts can be tailored to dancing seated on a chair, dancing in a pool, dancing for kids or for moms with their babies. As Bessie said, "Variety is the spice of life."

What are the health benefits of Zumba?

Zumba mixes low-intensity and high-intensity moves for an interval-style calorie-burning workout. It's a total body workout combining all elements of fitness: cardio, muscle conditioning, balance, and flexibility. So many people have had huge successes in losing unwanted pounds and inches, and reducing their body-fat percentages. Zumba is also an exhilarating feel-good workout that will boost your energy levels. Not only will you improve your body but your mood will get a boost too. You will feel amazing!

Am I too old for Zumba?

Nope! Zumba classes are tailored for all ages and all levels. There are specific Zumba class formats available based on the intensity desired. There's something for every body!

How do I get started?

It's easy! Find a comfortable pair of sneakers you can dance in. Bring some water. Get ready for an awesome workout! Relax and shake that bum to the music!

CROSSFIT

Ever seen a group of people flipping tractor tires down the sidewalk? They're not crazy, they're flipping their way to better fitness! But tires are just one part of CrossFit training, so don't let that scare you off. CrossFit is one of the fastest-growing workout programs in the United States, and it might be right for the fitness warrior in you! I talked CrossFit with Lisa Davis, host of the radio show *It's Your Health,* to get the full rundown.

What is CrossFit?

CrossFit is a whole-body workout that combines functional movement with high intensity—and even if you're fit, it can be a tough workout! It is definitely scalable to each person's fitness level, so start slow and easy, and work your way up.

What are the health benefits of CrossFit?

CrossFit workouts have been shown to have a positive effect on bone density as we age, along with keeping the central nervous system sharp and increasing muscle mass and strength. They incorporate the use of one's own body weight (gymnastic movements, running, jumping), barbells, dumbbells, kettlebells, medicine balls, Olympic weight lifting, and strongman training. Due to their high metabolic demand, CrossFit workouts increase EPOC (excess post-exercise oxygen consumption), enabling one to burn more calories at rest.

Another positive aspect of CrossFit is the fact that each and every workout has the potential to be quite different from the last, which some find to be mentally challenging. For many people, this tends to keep things fun and interesting, which may increase their motivation and desire to stick with it.

Am I too old for CrossFit?

As with most of the exercises we've discussed, it depends on the class. CrossFit workouts can be very challenging and the quick movements, if not properly done, can easily lead to injury. Pushing yourself too hard can also lead to overexercising or injury, so make sure to monitor your progress and build up your workouts slowly.

How do I get started?

Do some research online and find a class nearby. You'll want to start at a beginner level to learn all of the specific moves first. You'll be setting goals, and breaking them, in no time!

BELLY DANCING

Still have a dancing itch that Zumba didn't scratch? Try belly dancing. Ivette Oliveras, a teacher at Serena Studios in New York City, explained to me how belly dancing can put the spice back into boring workout routines.

What is belly dancing?

Belly dancing, also known as *raqs sharqi,* is a form of dance that uses graceful hip drops, rolls, and pivots, which utilize muscle groups in the abdomen, pelvis, trunk, spine, and neck. Belly dancing is quite popular as a form of exercise because it is known to work *with* the body instead of *against* it and is based on movements that come naturally to the female form.

What are the health benefits of belly dancing?

Belly dancing helps create a strong core, improves joint flexibility, encourages deeper breathing, and reduces stress. It's an aerobic workout that burns fat, raises metabolism, improves resting heart rate, tones major muscle groups, and even prepares major muscle groups for childbirth.

Am I too old for belly dancing?

Belly dancing is appropriate for all ages and helps women explore their femininity. It is a low-impact workout that promotes a strong core and healthy hips.

How do I get started?

Get a belly dancing hip scarf, find a class or online video, and just go for it! Recruit a friend to come along with you if you're nervous about attending a class alone.

Working out is not just about going to the gym—your options are endless! I hope the suggestions I laid out here and have explored on the show have inspired you to start looking for classes and programs that are available in your area. Go ahead and try them all—you are sure to find the fitness routine that works for your lifestyle.

If you can't find a class, there are endless free online videos of great ten- to sixty-minute workouts, available right at your fingertips. Find one you love or combine several for a workout tailored to your needs and goals. Here are some ideas to get you started:

- **PopSugar:** Check out the ten-minute workouts—perfect for the busy woman! (www.popsugar.com/workouts)

- **Blogilates:** Cassey Ho's Lean Legs Workout is a killer! (www.youtube.com/user/blogilates)

- **BeFit:** (www.youtube.com/user/BeFit)

I've also heard great things about former dancer Mary Helen Bower's Ballet Beautiful from my model friends. Her website is www .balletbeautiful.com.

Ask Carol

I absolutely hate cardio—running, biking, and so on. Any suggestions?

ANSWER:

Try a rebounder! A rebounder, or mini trampoline, offers so many health benefits, starting with its being a low-impact cardio workout. Rebounding boosts lymphatic drainage and improves digestion and balance—it's a full-body detox and so much more. I've never had so much fun during a cardio workout. I suggest purchasing

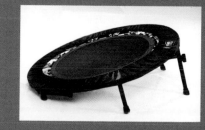

a rebounder so you can periodically do this workout over and over. But if you don't want to invest in one, call your local gym to see if they have one, or try a rebounder class.

The Power of Stretching

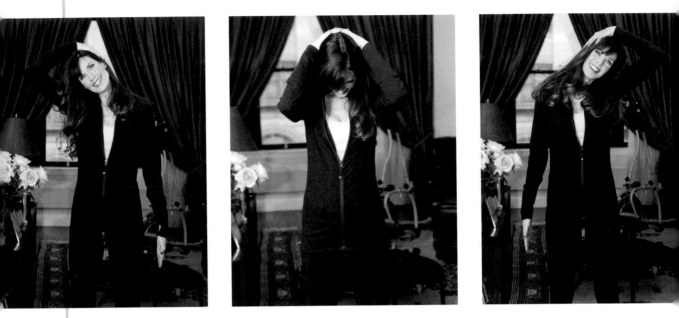

OK, so you carved out time in your crazy day and went to that Zumba class. Good job! You completed the first part of the battle and made your health a priority. There's one more step in your full fitness plan, though: stretching. Instead of racing out the door after a good workout, it's important you take time to stretch. People often quickly stretch their hamstrings or quads as they make for the parking lot, or they just skip this step altogether. Stretching is extremely important—especially as you age! Doctors, chiropractors, and physical therapists all agree that it's an important part of keeping your body fit. Flexibility is the third pillar of fitness, next to cardiovascular conditioning and strength training.

When you are young, it's so easy to touch your toes—who thinks twice about it? But as you age, if you don't stretch daily, doing basic tasks that require flexibility gets a lot tougher. Those shoelaces aren't going to tie themselves, so let's get stretching!

I sat down with BJ Dowlen, president of Bodyworks Enterprises (or should I say, squatted down with BJ), to talk stretching. She taught me an interesting fact—in Asian countries like Japan, people don't have as many hip surgeries as we do in the United States. Some think it's because other cultures squat more—to eat meals (at low tables), to use bathrooms, and so on. The simple act of squatting down to the floor daily can help your hips stay flexible.

WHY IS IT IMPORTANT TO STRETCH?

Stretching does so much and takes so little time. A simple daily stretching routine can:

- Decrease your risk of injury while working out
- Increase your range of motion in your joints
- Improve your posture
- Increase your blood circulation
- Increase your energy levels
- Reduce muscle tension
- Reduce inflammation
- Improve your balance
- Improve your mental focus

Not convinced yet? For women, stretching has also been known to reduce period pain.

Even though most of us have been stretching since elementary school gym class, BJ is often asked the same few questions about correct stretching techniques. Let's set the record straight!

SHOULD YOU STRETCH BEFORE EXERCISE?

No, your body is not warmed up yet. Instead, you should warm up for your exercise by doing dynamic movements, which mimic the moves of your workout, but at a lower intensity. Some suggestions are a brisk walk, walking lunges, leg swings, jumping jacks, high steps, or butt kicks for five to seven minutes.

SHOULD YOU STRETCH AFTER EXERCISE?

This is the best time to stretch, as your body will get the most benefit from a post-workout stretch session. You are more flexible after exercise because you have increased the circulation to your muscles and joints.

Dr. David Kulla, a chiropractor and the owner of Synergy Wellness Chiropractic & Physical Therapy in New York City, suggests these additional stretching tips:

- Never compare your flexibility with anyone else's, and stay within your comfort range. Your range will increase as you stretch more frequently and consistently.

- Some sensations you may feel during a stretch range from warmth in the muscle to a burning sensation or even sharp pain. If a stretch becomes painful or the discomfort is too strong—back off and do not continue. Do not push your end range of motion and never hold an intense stretch for longer than fifteen seconds.

- Don't bounce! Bouncing causes microtrauma in the muscle, which heals with scar tissue and will make you less flexible in the end.

- Always bend forward after bending backward because the muscles in the spine tend to tighten when going backward.

- It is better to hold a stretch at different angles for a short duration rather than holding one angle for a long period of time. The more intense the stretch, the shorter the duration you should hold it.

- Never hold your breath. It's extremely important to breathe while stretching. This allows your muscles to relax and get the most out of the stretch.

- Over time, slumping over and not sitting up straight can cause your muscles to shorten. (Similarly, wearing high heels causes shortening of the calf muscles because the shoes put them in a perpetual state of contraction.)

- *Don't* stretch first thing in the morning, especially if you have a low-back injury. Wait at least a half hour after you wake. While you sleep, your spine swells with fluid because of gravity, and the heaviest part of the body, the torso, usually sags lowest on a mattress, especially a soft one. This is why a more supportive firm mattress is recommended for people with back problems.

- *Don't* stretch the muscles you're about to train, as stretching tends to relax muscles. Research has shown doing so will decrease both strength and power. Although you should always warm up prior to an activity, stretching before one may actually cause injuries, not prevent them.

- *Don't* stretch if you are already very flexible! There is really no benefit to going too far to any extreme. Overstretching already flexible muscles can actually promote joint laxity and instability.

Follow these helpful tips to maximize your muscles' potential and get the most out of your stretching.

The Busy Woman's Fitness Plan

What is the most common excuse I hear when it comes to exercise? "I don't have time." I've used it. We've all used it. I get it! It can seem overwhelming to add in exercise when your day already feels packed to the brim.

We all lead busy lives. Even so, I strongly believe that it is essential to take time for self-care every day. Exercise is one of the most important things you can do for yourself, and your family, to ensure that you live a long, full, disease-free life.

There must be a solution to get over this common setback. I spoke with Michael Roberts, executive editor of *Outside* magazine, who has interviewed top executives about this very question of time management. How are busy industry leaders able to balance a satisfying family life with working out? Here's how they do it:

- Be efficient. Make every minute of your day count.

- Multitask and find ways to exercise in your daily life—even at work. (We have you covered! Read on for Tony Greco's Five-Minute Exercises for Everyone, page 137, and a series of exercises you can do at home or work, page 142.)

- Set fitness goals and stick to them.

- Find someone to work out with.

- Eat smarter. You won't be able to properly work out or be fit if you don't fuel your body correctly.

As I said earlier, there is no magic diet or fitness plan! The tips offered in this part of the book should help to remind you that fitness needs to be a priority, one that you commit to fully. It's not always about time spent—it's about maximizing your efforts! Setting goals, finding a workout buddy, setting aside uninterrupted workout time—these strategies can all help you to hold yourself accountable.

Five-Minute Exercises for Everyone

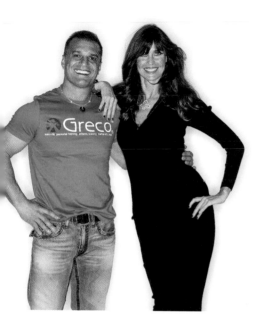

Still feel like you don't have time? Tony Greco, owner of Greco Fitness, who works with celebrities like Carrie Underwood (have you seen her legs?), shared a few easy, no-gym-needed exercises with me. No more excuses! If you would like a visual to follow these exercises, head to my blog at www.carolalt.com or use this link: bit.ly/CA_5MinExercise.

ROTATION LUNGE WITH WATER JUG

Preparation: Stand with your legs hip distance apart.

Execution: Shift your weight onto your left leg, pivot on your right foot, and lower your body into a lunge as you simultaneously rotate your torso and the water jug to the left. Repeat for 30 seconds, then switch legs.

SINGLE LEG SQUAT PICKING UP A CONE

Preparation: Stand with your feet shoulder width apart. Balance on one leg with the opposite knee bent and raised at a 90-degree angle. (You can use a chair for balance.) Set a cone, block, or water bottle in front of you.

Execution: Squat down as far as possible while keeping your bent knee off the floor. Keep your back straight and your supporting knee pointed in the same direction as the foot supporting it. Bend over, grab the cone, and stand back up. Do 30 seconds on one leg and then repeat with the other.

CROSS OVER THE DUCT TAPE

Preparation: Stick a 5-foot length of duct tape on the floor. Start at one end of the tape you set up.

Execution: Moving sideways, lift your trailing leg over your lead leg with each step in a grapevine motion. Repeat back and forth over the duct tape. Can be done anywhere.

THE BIRD DOG

The Bird Dog yoga pose strengthens your abs and lower back and butt muscles while improving your balance.

1. **Starting position:** Come to a hands and knees position on an exercise mat, positioning your knees underneath your hips and the crease of your wrists directly underneath your shoulders. Your fingers should be pointing forward.

2. **Engage your core and abdominal muscles:** Imagine you are tightening a corset around your waistline. Keep your spine in a neutral position, avoid any excessive sagging or arching. Pull your shoulder blades toward your hips.

3. **Upward phase:** In this exercise you are attempting to move the opposite arm and leg simultaneously. It is very helpful to use a mirror to help with form adjustments. Begin by slowly raising the left leg until it is long and strong, and parallel or nearly parallel to the floor. The leg should not be lifted above hip height. This will help to avoid upward rotation at the hip.

4. **Slowly raise and straighten your right arm:** Attempt to raise the arm until it is parallel to the floor. Do not allow the shoulders to tilt upward. Keep them parallel to the floor. Your head is an extension of your spine and should remain aligned with the spine throughout the movement. Do not lift the head or let it sag downward.

   NOTE: The leg and arm should only be raised to heights that allow you to keep the shoulders and pelvis parallel, the core engaged, and the spine in neutral position.

5. **Downward phase:** Gently lower back to the starting position, maintaining balance and stability in the shoulders, pelvis, and torso.

6. **Alternating sides:** During this phase of changing sides, work very hard to keep the abdominals engaged. Imagine that your ribs are being knit together as though you were lacing up a tennis shoe. When you change sides, try to do so with minimal weight shift. Do not flop from one side to the next. Maintain balance and control.

Perform each exercise for 1 minute and then rest for 30 seconds. Repeat each exercise five times for a total time of 5 minutes of work a day. To burn even more fat, add cardiovascular exercises like walking, biking, jogging, or running for another 20 to 30 minutes.

You don't need to spend hours at the gym—you just need to be doing the correct movements to get results. Take the time to set yourself up for success.

Stand Up to Sitting Down

In modern society, most of us tend to spend the majority of our day sitting. We spend countless hours in front of a computer screen or at a desk and then go home and sit on the couch after a long, stressful day. This type of sedentary lifestyle is not healthy and leads to disease and health issues.

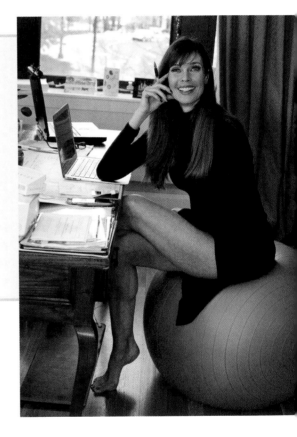

Carol's Tip

I spend a lot of time in my office and in front of a computer too! I bought one of those exercise balls, which has helped a lot with my posture and keeping me grounded. If you have to sit all day, you should try to find ways to be active every hour!

According to the American Heart Association, "sedentary jobs have increased 83% since 1950. Physically active jobs now make up only about 25% of our workforce, which is 50% less than 1950." I had Dr. Florence Comite, a top Manhattan endocrinologist and leader in the emerging field of precision medicine, on my show to discuss the effects of a sedentary lifestyle. Dr. Comite explained that a sedentary lifestyle increases your chance of gaining weight and developing a number of chronic diseases, such as heart disease, diabetes, high blood pressure, certain cancers, stroke, sleep apnea, osteoarthritis, and even infertility. The good news? We can reverse this course easily! Dr. Comite suggested getting up from your computer and walking around or stretching every twenty to thirty minutes. She also suggested incorporating extra activity whenever possible—taking the stairs to your next meeting instead of the elevator or pacing during a phone call. Even fidgeting helps! You can also try active sitting, using an exercise ball or a dynamic chair that engages the core, an under-the-desk pedal exerciser, or use a standing desk during your workday. Small lifestyle tweaks will help to reenergize the body and recharge the mind.

Let's stand up to sitting down! While you probably can't run out and quit your desk job tomorrow, you can take small steps toward making regular physical activity a priority in your day-to-day life. Just walking a short distance to fill your water bottle, taking a break while standing, or sneaking out for a lap around the block can break up long stretches of sitting down. Dr. Comite also recommends including a mixture of aerobic exercise, weight training, and restorative exercise during the week. These steps add up to a healthier, happier you by increasing your vitality and improving your health.

Fitness expert Jaime Morales shared with me some easy exercises you can do at your desk or in a break or conference room. If you want additional visuals, head to my blog at www.carolalt.com or this link: bit.ly/CA_DeskExercises.

All of these exercises require only your desk chair (one with no wheels!).

Carol's Tip

I keep my yoga mat in a place where it stares me down and beckons me to work out—right in front of my desk. And after a workout, it sits there and congratulates me!

PLANK TWISTS

Start on a basic forearm plank with straight legs. Start by bending and twisting your left knee toward the right side of the chair. Hold for 2 seconds before going back to the starting position. Keep switching legs for 30 seconds, while keeping your focus on control, posture, and length.

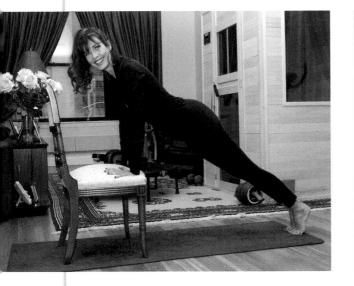 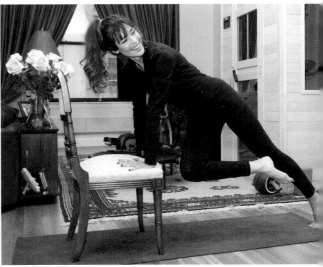

ALTERNATING SIDE PLANKS

Start on a basic forearm plank with straight legs. Lift and turn your body into a side plank. From there, kick the top leg up from your outer thighs. Drop the leg and go back to regular plank. Alternate sides. Focus on relaxing your neck while keeping a straight spin and straight legs.

TRICEPS DIPS

Start sitting on the edge of an office chair with your hands next to your hips and your shoulders back. Lift your hips and slowly lower your body close to the floor, bending your elbows back. Hold the down position for 5 seconds, focusing mostly on keeping your elbows in toward each other and relaxing the neck and shoulders. Press back up while squeezing the triceps. Try doing 10 to 15 repetitions with perfect form.

PUSH-UPS

Start on a long arm plank (the push-up position) with good body posture and hands under shoulders. Slowly lower your body as far down as possible without losing control. Hold for a second before pushing yourself back to start.

ONE-LEG DEAD-LIFTS

Stand on one leg, with your opposite leg in front of or behind you. With good posture, hinge forward from the hips, sticking your butt out and feeling strength and length from the back of your working leg. Hold the bent-over position for 2 to 4 seconds before coming back to standing. Repeat 10 to 15 times and then switch legs.

Carol's Tip

Conference calls are my favorite time to get a workout in! If I'm just listening in, I start doing squats or bounce on my rebounder. It's a great time to exercise-multitask.

Proper Posture

Did you know that standing up straight can visually take up to 10 pounds of body weight off your frame? It's true! Good posture is an excellent way to improve the way you look, but looking tall and attractive isn't the only reason to work on how you stand and sit—there's far more to it than that. Good posture influences a number of things—your risk of experiencing lower back pain, your energy levels, your focus, and your concentration. If you're constantly in a slouched position all day, there's far less oxygen coming into the body. Low levels of oxygen are one of the contributing factors to fatigue.

Good posture also means your bones are properly aligned and your muscles, joints, and ligaments can work as nature intended. Your vital organs will be in the right position and can function at peak efficiency. Good posture also contributes to the normal functioning of the nervous system.

Without good posture, your overall health and total efficiency may be compromised. The long-term effects of poor posture can involve many bodily systems (such as digestion, elimination, breathing), muscles, joints, and ligaments, so it's so important to focus on your posture and correct any bad habits!

WHAT CAUSES BAD POSTURE?

One of the top offenders: bad work ergonomics.

We spend so much time at our desks that small bad habits can build up over time and lead to major posture problems. If your desk or chair isn't set at the right height for you, you won't be able to sustain good posture throughout the day. I use a balance ball as my chair at my desk to help my posture!

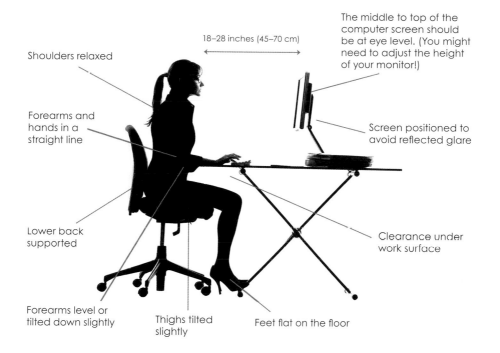

Shoulders relaxed

18–28 inches (45–70 cm)

The middle to top of the computer screen should be at eye level. (You might need to adjust the height of your monitor!)

Forearms and hands in a straight line

Screen positioned to avoid reflected glare

Lower back supported

Clearance under work surface

Forearms level or tilted down slightly

Thighs tilted slightly

Feet flat on the floor

I talked to Dr. David Kulla, owner of Synergy Wellness in New York City, and got his best advice on maintaining good posture while you sit.

I learned that another bad habit that leads to poor posture is not moving enough during the day. The more you sit for long periods of time, the greater the chances that you aren't using good posture. Breaking up your day with activity allows you to stand upright more often. This decreases the amount of compression stress that's put on your spinal column.

Finally, the last bad habit that leads to poor posture is overtraining your chest muscles without enough focus on the back muscles. It's important to develop good balance between chest and back training. If you lift weights, make sure to work out evenly. This can even happen in yoga as you are using your front muscles, for poses like Chaturanga, and not your back. If the chest becomes overly strong, it will start to pull your shoulders forward. This creates a rounded appearance where your shoulders are caving in.

GOOD POSTURE AND AGING

As you age, your posture becomes more and more important. Don't just take my word for it. According to Dr. Kulla, poor posture can:

- **Limit your range of motion.** Muscles can be permanently shortened or stretched when a slumped-over position becomes your normal position. Muscles and ligaments that have been shortened or stretched no longer function as they should.

- **Increase discomfort and pain.** Bad posture resulting from a forward-head position can often cause headaches and pain in the shoulders, arms, hands, and around the eyes. Rounded shoulders can trigger headaches at the base of your skull where the shoulder muscles attach.

- **Create pain in the jaw.** A forward-head position can lead to jaw pain known as temporomandibular joint disease (TMJ) that was once considered only a dental problem. Today we know that TMJ-related pain also may be caused or aggravated by faulty posture.

- **Decrease lung capacity.** Reducing the amount of oxygen in your body can decrease the space in your chest cavity, restricting efficient functioning of your lungs.

- **Cause lower back pain.** This is one of the most common consequences of bad posture. For people over thirty-five, lower back pain is often interpreted as a sure sign of age, although it may have been developing since childhood.

- **Cause nerve interference.** Your spine is the basis of posture. If your posture is bad, your spine can be misaligned. Spinal misalignments may cause interference in nerve function.

- **Affect proper bowel function.** Even this important bodily task may be affected by faulty posture. If you have a rounded shoulders, head-forward posture, it may affect your bowels. If your spine arches and sways forward, your intestines may sag, which causes constipation.

- **Make you look older than you are.** When you are slumped, hunched over, or not standing straight, you can add years to your appearance. For women, the more rounded the shoulders, the more breasts may sag. Any woman, no matter what her age, can help reduce the sag in her breasts by nearly 50 percent by simply standing tall.

IMPROVING YOUR POSTURE

It's pretty simple to improve your posture; you just need to be more conscious of it on a daily basis. When standing, hold your head high, point your chin firmly forward and parallel to the earth, push your shoulders back and your chest out, and tuck your stomach in to increase your balance. Here are some other specific ways to improve your posture throughout your day:

- If you stand all day in a job like a cashier or clerk, rest one foot on a stool and take breaks to get off your feet for a while.

- Spending a lot of time sitting at a desk every day can wreak havoc on your body. Make sure to stand up every 15 to 30 minutes and stretch. Bend over and incorporate exercises, like the ones on page 142, into your desk routine.

- When sitting in the car for a long period, you should adjust the seat forward so your knees are higher than your hips. Put a small pillow or cushion behind the small of your back.

- When sleeping you should lie on your side with your knees bent and head supported by a pillow to make your head level with your spine. Or sleep on your back, avoiding thick pillows under your head. Use a small pillow under your neck instead. Try to avoid sleeping on your stomach.

- When bending, never twist from the waist and bend forward at the same time. To lift or reach something on the floor, bend the knees while keeping the back straight.

If you follow these practices, but still feel discomfort and pain related to specific activities, you should consider visiting a chiropractor for a checkup and a postural evaluation.

Ask Carol

I sit at a computer all day, with everything set up ergonomically, but I still find myself slumping over my computer screen. Any other tips?

ANSWER:

I had Owen McKibbin, an ambassador for the AlignMed Posture Shirt, as a guest on *A Healthy You & Carol Alt*. He introduced me to the shirt, which uses cutting-edge technology to create neuro bands that help with muscle mapping to improve posture, relieve pain, increase balance and flexibility, reduce fatigue, and improve recovery rate. The shirt helps pull your shoulders back and down, while opening your chest. It can be found at www.alignmed.com. If you're on a budget, there's also a less expensive version from Back Joy that I've heard great things about. You can get it from www.backjoy.com.

Mindful Meditation

We live in an age of constant motion. I can't tell you how many of my friends tell me how busy they are all of the time! Every day we rush to try to get as much done as humanly possible. With smartphones and tablets connected to our hands, we spend so much time planning out our next steps, next day, week, and even year. While we seem to be maximizing our time, be it at work, at home, with friends or family, this type of go-go-go lifestyle also has its drawbacks.

We often forget to enjoy the present moment—to stop and reflect how wonderful it is to simply breathe and be alive. I had the pleasure of having Russell Simmons, best known as the cofounder of Def Jam records, on my show. He is currently going across America promoting meditation in schools. Russell wrote a wonderful book, *Success Through Stillness,* which chronicles his experience with meditation and helps guide readers to use stillness as a powerful tool to fully access their potential.

Russell stumbled into meditation after attending a yoga class filled with "beautiful women" fifteen years ago. In *Success Through Stillness,* he shows the connection between inner peace and outward success. Russell believes his meditation practice changed his life for the better and says that there is no bad way to meditate, only different forms for different people.

Many people have misconceptions about meditation. You don't have to be a Buddhist or Tibetan monk and you don't have to go to India to learn how to be present and meditate. Meditation can actually stimulate your mind to be more creative and industrious. A little break during the day can reap big benefits! Meditation can help in many physical, psychological, and spiritual ways:

- Meditation helps reduce stress and tension (by teaching you how to "switch off" your mind).

- It helps lower blood pressure.

- It may slow down aging.

- It helps you learn how to control your thoughts (increases self-awareness).

- It helps you enjoy subtle things in life (scents, breathing, being).

- It can improve your mental focus, concentration, and creativity.

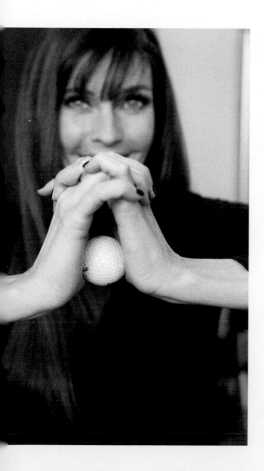

Carol's Tip

My favorite stress-reduction technique is from Barbara Kunz, author of *Complete Reflexology for Life*.

Barbara and her husband, Kevin, are the most knowledgeable reflexologists I know! They taught me two great tricks to reduce stress using just a golf ball. Barbara suggests clasping your fingers together with the ball to massage the pads of your hands. I love this! Kevin recommends keeping a golf ball under your desk to roll beneath your feet for an instant massage. When I get stressed I take a minute to lightly roll my feet, stimulating the Vagus nerve, which is on the ball of your foot between the big toe and the second toe. It's an anti-aging trick that's actually supposed to make you look younger. Give it a try!

A SIMPLE WAY TO START MEDITATING

1. Make the time! Set aside 10 to 15 minutes for yourself. I like to do this before I go to bed, but many people enjoy it when they first wake up.

2. Set yourself in a comfortable position in a quiet and relaxing area. I like to sit with my legs crossed in front of me, my palms resting on my legs and facing the ceiling.

3. Close your eyes and concentrate on your breath. This was hard for me! I couldn't shut off what Russell called my Monkey Mind. The Monkey Mind describes the mind when you try to cage it. It becomes like a monkey, jumping all over from this thought to that thought. I would try not to think, which, in turn, would cause me to think of everything! If you run into this problem, too, remember to try not to cage your mind. Relax with your thoughts, start counting your breaths, or choose a mantra to repeat. It could be something simple like "I am at peace. I am at peace." Say it over and over. Keep at it—the more you practice meditation, the easier it becomes.

4. Enjoy these moments and don't beat yourself up if you can't meditate for a long time—eventually you'll get it. It's important to take some time for yourself each day.

Now that you've heard me say it throughout this section, you can't possibly ignore it—you need to exercise! It is essential to having a long, happy, healthy life. I've now armed you with some specific ways you can partake in physical activity, as well as with a better understanding of just how many health benefits come with regular exercise. Hopefully it will be harder for you to fall back on those excuses now! The hardest part, for most people, is simply putting on your shoes and getting your butt in gear to go to a class or activity. I have a yoga teacher who starts each class by saying, "Congratulations. You are here and have already done 50 percent of the work!" Each time you lace up and head out the door, remind yourself that you are taking care of your body and that you should soon begin to feel, look, and sleep a lot better!

PART 3

Skin Care & Beauty

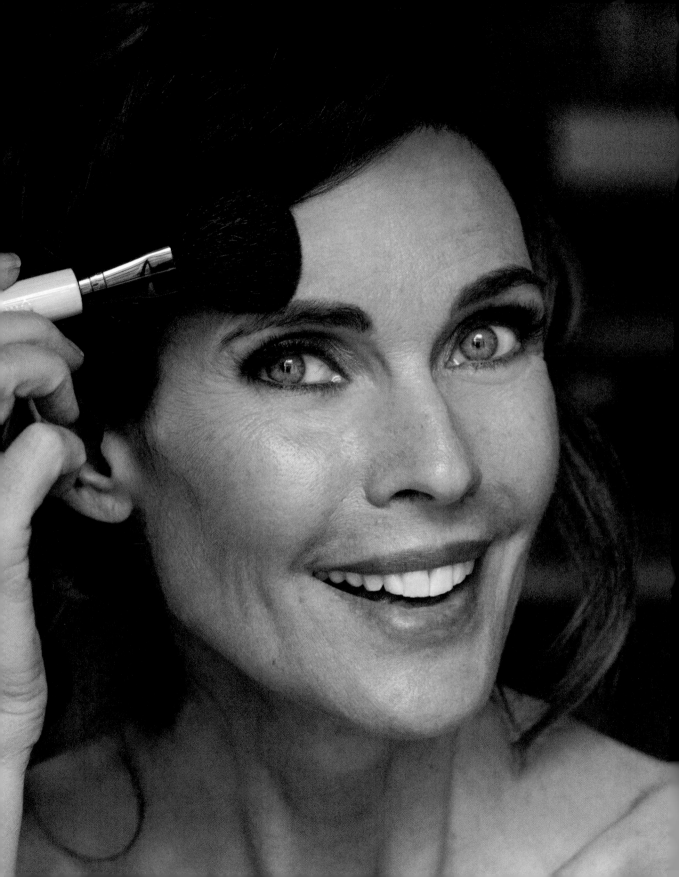

*I*f you flipped right to this section because you want my best beauty advice, or to learn more about the products and makeup that I use, you are missing out on some of the most valuable beauty secrets in this book: good nutrition and regular exercise! If you don't practice self-care and make an effort to show your body some love by eating well and exercising, then nothing I can tell you in this next section will matter. A healthy lifestyle is the foundation of my beauty routine and should be the most important part of yours.

As a model, and now as a television host, I've always had to focus on my outer beauty as part of my day-to-day job. During my many years in front of the camera I've had the opportunity to work with fabulous hair and makeup teams, dermatologists, and talented stylists and designers, and I've learned so many tricks of the trade when it comes to beauty and fashion. While I could fill a whole other book with quick tips and lists of the best products, my advice on beauty and fashion is much simpler.

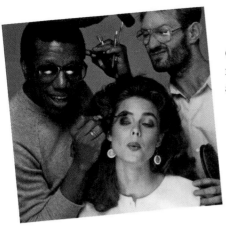

Goofing on the set with makeup artist Joey Mills and hairstylist Alex.

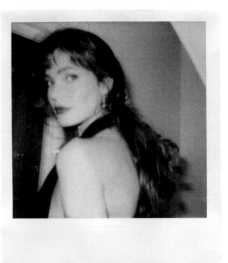

A snapshot from 1990, on the set of the movie *Millions* with Billy Zane and Lauren Hutton.

I call this my half a cover—this is the twenty-fifth anniversary of the *Sports Illustrated* Swimsuit Edition. Kathy Ireland had the main cover, and all the original cover girls each got a supplementary cover.

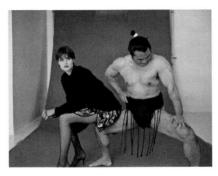

I shot this photo for Italian *Vogue*. The sumo wrestler came in that morning and slammed his feet on the floor—the whole building shook!

With photographer Claude Mougin *(right)* and his assistant *(left)*. We were just having fun, mugging for the camera.

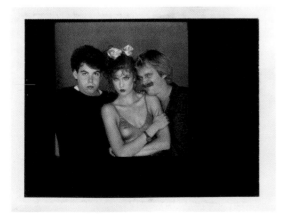

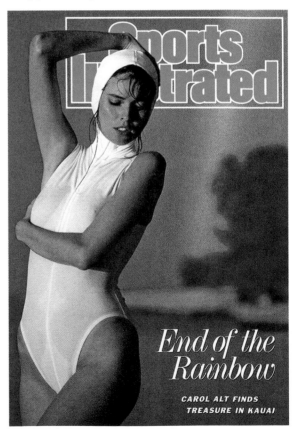

True beauty is not only about how you look on the outside—it's also your inner self. Beauty stems from the kind of life you live and the choices, both big and small, that you make every day. I believe that if you choose to nurture your body by eating well and exercising, it will show in every way—your weight, your skin, your self-confidence, your attitude, and your energy. In my fifties, I am now finally at a point in my life where everything is falling into place because I have learned to love and take care of my body. You only have one body—treat it right!

My friend and makeup artist Carmindy, from TLC's *What Not to Wear,* said it best: "What truly makes a woman beautiful is what she radiates from within and then cares for on the outside. It's an absolute confidence and self-love that shines from the soul into other people's eyes. It moves you. It transforms you. It's contagious. I call it 'soul beauty.'"

Beauty isn't about a one-size-fits-all routine or expensive products—it's more about a feeling and attitude. It's about owning and celebrating your uniqueness. When I was younger, I always felt awkward about being nearly six feet tall. My sister Karen was also very tall but very thin, and people called her "Twiggy"; they sarcastically called me "Twig-let" because I was tall, too, but nowhere near as thin as my sister. I wasted precious time worrying and feeling self-conscious about my height, which was something I couldn't change but was also a feature that actually became an advantage when I began modeling. Over time, I learned to love my height; it was part of what made me special, part of my beauty, and I could spend my time slouching to fit in or I could choose to embrace it and show it off to the world. I chose the latter and have never looked back! After all, my height was the catalyst for my modeling career and became one of the reasons I had the opportunity to write this book.

We live in a society where people are bombarded by Photoshopped photographs at every turn. We can't help but compare ourselves with an unrealistic portrayal of beauty. Growing up in the modeling industry, I was a part of that illusion, but it was a different time. Sure, we had our

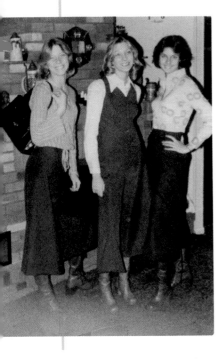

Christmas Day 1985—the beginning of my modeling career! *From left to right:* my younger sister, Christine; my older sister, Karen; and me. (Karen made the gauchos!)

tricks in the 1980s, but airbrushing wasn't done to the extent it is today. When I first started modeling there wasn't a size 00. You had to be thin, fit, and in shape, but it was nothing like the thin that's in today. A few years ago, I was at a show during Fashion Week and my friend, who was the designer, said to me, "Oh my, that model walking the runway is skin and bones. I felt so bad, I had to hire her." This comment flabbergasted me—hire her just because she's starving herself for the job? I told him he was sending the wrong message. By using a model who looked unhealthy, he set an impossible standard for every other model whom he didn't hire. It was spreading the already dangerous message that thinner equals better. In the past few years, I've been very proud of companies like Dove and Aerie that are breaking the mold and have used strong and untouched models for their campaigns. Even companies like Victoria's Secret, which every top model aspires to work with, are pushing for strong and toned women instead of just skinny ones.

Today, I always request that photos of me not be retouched. I want women to see firsthand the power of raw food and a healthy lifestyle, and the only way I can do that is to walk the walk. Women should feel sexy as they age, but again and again the media tries to make them feel like they need to have work done, or have their photos touched up. I feel more confident than ever at this point in my life and I want the world to see it—laugh lines and all!

In this part I want to look at both inner and outer beauty—especially how feeling more confident in your own skin and celebrating your uniqueness benefits your body and soul. Then we'll dive into the skin care and beauty tips that will keep you looking and feeling radiant today and for many years to come.

Is Beauty Skin Deep?

I love working with makeup artist Carmindy, because instead of trying to make you look "perfect," she believes in celebrating your uniqueness. My eyes are one of my favorite features, so she always makes sure to use special touches to make them stand out. Carmindy believes in making you look like the best version of you—something I support wholeheartedly. Her most recent book, *Bloom: A Girl's Guide to Growing Up,* offers this positive message to teens. I'm so glad. It's important for women of all ages to hear it!

Here are Carmindy's five tips on how to harness your inner soul beauty and let it shine for the whole world to see!

1. Practice Mirror Mantras

The first thing you must learn to do is to turn off any negative, broken-record, self-hate thoughts. This might take some time as you are proba-

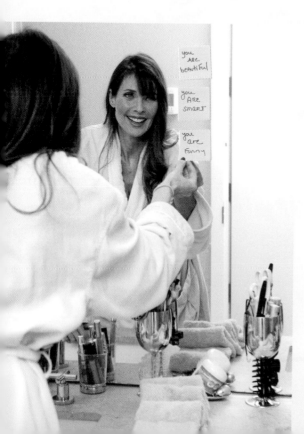

bly breaking an old habit, so it won't happen overnight. It takes practice!

Each time a nasty thought like "My eyes are so tiny" crosses your mind, you should instantly look into the mirror and follow up the negative thought with a positive one like "I love my sweet smile." When you say these positive words into the mirror each day, you will be on your way to a new path of beauty enlightenment. It might seem silly at first, but it will get easier and easier as you retrain your brain. You can even write a mantra on your mirror each day or program an alert into your smartphone as a reminder of your awesomeness.

Carol's Tip

The mirror can be your friend, projecting back at you the most beautiful parts of yourself! Instead of picking apart one feature you dislike, focus on another you love.

2. Let Go

This next step is an important one. In order to unleash your soul beauty, you need to face your past. Start by doing some searching inside. When you identify the source of your insecurities and pain you can allow your soul to face the issue, forgive it, and let it go once and for all.

Even many years after the fact, you might still be holding on to painful memories about your appearance. Maybe kids made fun of you for being overweight in school, or an overbearing parent criticized the way you looked, or an abusive boyfriend or husband said hurtful things to you. It could even be your own inner self that is constantly critiquing your outer beauty. It is time for peace.

I want you to get to a quiet place, whether through meditation, going for a long walk, or even taking a hot bath. Now face that dark place you've identified and breathe deeply. I want you to acknowledge that you, at this moment and forever, are filled with a pure beautiful light that glows from within. It is never again going to be diminished or dimmed. Take your power back! Own your uniqueness and understand that you are special, important, and beautiful. Know that the person or people who have hurt you are just coming from a fearful and hurt place themselves. Forgive them as you breathe in, and as you breathe out let go of those negative memories. Love yourself. That is the true secret of the most confident, self-assured, and happy people in the world.

3. Practice the Ancient Feminine Ritual of Beautification

For thousands of years women have enhanced their looks—from Egyptians lining their eyes to the ancient Mesopotamians wearing lipstick. The main difference between our female ancestors and us is that they used cosmetics for empowerment, while many of us are using them out of insecurity. Our ancestors used makeup to attract wealth, fertility, and love, and to ward off evil, create magic, and celebrate their lives. We use it to cover up flaws.

Some women skip makeup altogether because they feel it's selfish to take time out every day to pamper themselves. Taking care of your outer beauty is as important as taking care of your inner beauty, and you deserve it. If you enjoy wearing makeup, it's not selfish to take the time you need to take care of yourself. Taking five to ten minutes each day to enhance your natural beauty will not only empower you, but you will feel amazing and on top of your game. You don't need a multistep routine; just use the right products in the right places to play up your best features.

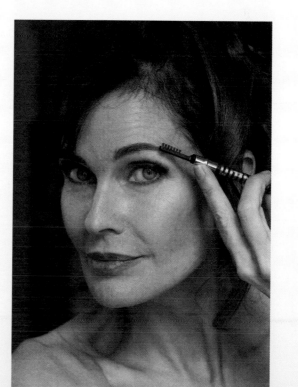

4. Feature Focus

An easy way to enhance your natural beauty is to play up your best features. I call it

Feature Focus. Instead of using cosmetics to change what you don't like about your face, use them to enhance what you love. Focus all that beautiful energy on the positive! Look into the mirror and kick away any corrosive thoughts. Try closing your eyes, breathing in, and saying, "I am beautiful." Now open your eyes. What lovely feature stands out to you? Is it a thick lash line? A cute splattering of freckles? A unique iris color? A quirky smile? Now use makeup to enhance that feature. Luscious lips can go bold with a fun new lipstick hue. Round cheeks can be celebrated with a highlighter and a swirl of pink blush. A strong nose can be accentuated with a shimmering face powder. Own your favorite features and focus on the beauty you possess.

5. Practice Contagious Compliments

It is our duty as women to help our fellow sisters feel strong and beautiful. We are living in a world where we see women tear each other down in reality shows and gossip in the workplace. I can't even begin to talk about all the bullying that goes on with our younger girls in school. Here's one solution—give a compliment and mean it. I promise, it will catch on! If we start practicing Contagious Compliments, we can start to change our collective consciousness, making us all feel confident and connected.

So next time you see a woman at the checkout counter at the grocery store with beautiful hair, tell her. If the bus driver has gorgeous skin, let her know. If your cousin's eyes are pretty, throw her a compliment. You never know what kind of day these women might be having, and chances are that you will make their day if you compliment them. It will make you feel good, too!

Thank you for these wonderful, life-changing tips, Carmindy! When you master these steps, your life will change. Your self-esteem will soar, you will attract abundance, and you will be truly beautiful— inside and out.

Carol's Tip

One of my favorite sayings is, "You don't have to blow out someone else's candle to make yours shine." In fact, I've found that every time I help someone else's light to shine, my own light shines even brighter!

How to Get Glowing Skin

What turns heads even more than a new dress or great makeup? Great skin. We know the basics of good skin: healthy eating and exercise. So now that we have our foundation, let's build up from there. Many people think that genetics is the main cause of good skin. According to my physician, Dr. Nicholas Gonzalez, having good genes doesn't hurt, but following good eating and health habits can make a world of difference to your skin. Beautiful skin is about practicing these good habits day in and day out. With our busy lives it's easy to forget to take care of ourselves, and our skin is the first to suffer the consequences: We don't eat correctly (and are missing those key raw building blocks). We fall asleep with makeup on, pop pimples, drink contaminated water, or use products that contain harmful ingredients because they are popular and advertised on television. This results in skin problems like wrinkles, acne, blackheads, dullness, and dryness.

Keep in mind, advertisers hire twenty- and thirty-year-olds to sell that antiwrinkle cream you saw on TV. Most of them, and I can say this from experience, don't even need the creams they are pushing. When I first started going raw, it was mainly for my health, but a wonderful side effect from my new diet was that my skin started looking better and better. I was in a competitive business where young girls were coming in every day and getting the best jobs. Because of the way I looked and felt before going raw, largely due to my poor diet, I thought my career was over at age thirty. How could I sell skin cream or shampoo as a spokesmodel when my hair looked terrible, my skin was already starting to wrinkle, and I was feeling sick all the time?

Once I changed my diet and went raw, people were shocked at how different I looked—and it happened so quickly! I got results immediately in terms of my health, and soon afterward (and I mean within days!), I had an outward change so significant that my friends commented about it in awe. I lost bloat and my skin glowed—and because I felt so happy and satisfied by being able to eat so guilt-free, I projected positivity and happiness. The great response I got from friends and colleagues alike bolstered my decision and gave me the confidence to continue down my raw food road. This is when I realized firsthand that no amount of wrinkle cream or makeup could help my skin if I didn't help it first through the food I was putting into my body. In fact, the makeup seemed to only enhance my issues, announcing to the world I had a pimple or that I had wrinkles.

My life-changing mantra? Change your food, change your looks.

After I changed my diet and nourished myself from the inside out, I needed the right beauty products and makeup to nourish my skin from the outside in. I did some research and realized that I could use quality foods as my external skin care also! Food-grade ingredients are always best for your beauty regime, because commercial products get diluted with so many questionable ingredients.

Carol's Tip

Smooth a couple of drops of olive oil over your face, elbows, and knees every day. Olive oil contains monounsaturated fat, which refreshes and hydrates skin without leaving a greasy feeling. Raw, unrefined coconut oil works great as well.

Here are skin care uses for some foods that you probably already have at home:

- Olive oil works as a natural eye makeup remover.

- Lemon juice can lighten dark spots on your skin. The juice helps to even color, but never go into the sunlight with it on, because it can cause your skin to burn.

- Coconut oil works to moisturize your skin. Carmindy puts hers in a jar in the refrigerator so it hardens, which makes it easier to handle as a moisturizer.

- Egg whites will seal and tighten your skin.

- Coffee grounds can be used to reduce puffiness. (Another use for coffee besides drinking it!)

I love food-based skin care so much I've included a whole section on it. See "Do It Yourself!" on page 186.

I turned to my friend, Marco Guidetti-Hoffman, founder of the Skin-Care Clinic of Switzerland, for some other tips on creating a natural glow.

1. DETOX

Detoxifying the skin helps it to glow. But I'm not talking about detoxing with a juice cleanse! Instead, the detox technique to use is called manual lymphatic massage (and Marco suggests getting two every year by a licensed massage therapist). This technique was invented by massage therapists Drs. Emil and Estrid Vodder and has been used since the early 1930s. This type of massage encourages the elimination of waste, helps improve the body's circulation, and benefits the muscular and nervous systems.

Encourage your massage therapist to focus on your neck, armpits, stomach, and the area behind the knees, as these are areas where there are a lot of lymph nodes. The lymphatic system is part of the body's defenses and removes microorganisms and other foreign substances. The lymph nodes act as a filtration system that keeps particulate matter, such as bacteria, from entering the bloodstream. Stimulating the nodes through manual lymphatic massages will also encourage fluid circulation and cell regeneration, which promote detoxification, facilitate healing, and support the immune system.

Who knew something so enjoyable could also be so good for you!

Two other ways to help detoxify your skin (that you can do in the comfort of your home) are to purchase a rebounder—which is also great for exercise!—and use a natural dry skin brush daily.

Carol's Tip

Skin brushing is an Ayurvedic practice that helps the body in many different ways, including stimulating lymphatic drainage (detox!), exfoliating the skin, and improving your circulation and the overall quality of your skin. Skin brushing should be done with a natural bristle skin brush on dry skin for about five minutes a day. You should always brush toward the heart, because that is the way the lymphatic system drains. Inexpensive dry skin brushes are sold online or at health-food stores.

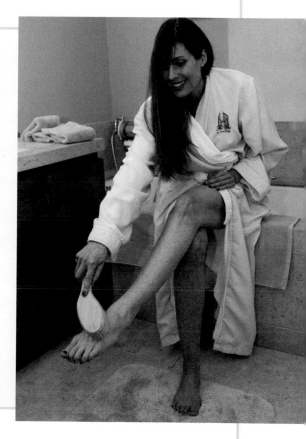

2. CLEANSE AND TONE

To keep skin looking fresh, plump, flexible, and dewy, be sure to cleanse every single morning and evening. Follow your cleansing routine by using a toner, and apply moisturizer to finish. Also, everyone should use a moisturizer that contains sunscreen. The sun is the worst aging force out there!

3. MAINTAIN THE "ENERGY" LEVEL OF THE SKIN TISSUE

A living skin cell requires energy, not only for all its functions, but also for the maintenance of its structure. If you don't sleep enough, or if you don't manage your stress, your skin won't have the energy it needs to properly repair itself and maintain its structure.

4. REVERSE SIGNS OF SUN DAMAGE

If you have sun damage, the most essential ingredients you should look for in your skin care products are retinoids. A licensed professional can usually recommend a retinol night serum for your skin type and condition (they come in different concentrations).

Carol's Tip

I love adding carrot seed essential oil to my skin-care regime because I feel it's perfect for anti-aging. It helps protect from environmental assaults such as pollution and stress, and may help reduce the appearance of wrinkles because carrot seed oil is high in antioxidants. Make sure you mix it with a base like olive oil or coconut oil. Don't use it straight on your skin.

5. USE TOPICAL ANTIOXIDANTS

Antioxidants, such as vitamins C and E, are proven to be beneficial for your skin, since they increase the protection power of sun-protective creams.

Carol's Tip

Skip long, steamy showers and instead opt for quicker, colder showers. Long, hot showers strip skin of its moisture and wash away protective oils. Cold showers are also great for your hair! And as a side benefit they kick your metabolism into gear—give it a try!

If you can't give up your hot shower, at least follow it by a blast of cold water. I laugh and scream in mine—yes, because it is cold. But it certainly wakes me up!

Are Your Makeup and Skin Care Products Aging You?

Most of us think of skin as just our body's visible outer layer, but it's actually our largest organ. Your skin absorbs everything you put on it. Just like the choices we make about what we put into our bodies for fuel, our choice of what we use on our bodies directly impacts our overall health.

According to the Environmental Working Group, a nonprofit organization focused on environment and public health, the average woman uses 12 beauty products per day, with a combined total of about 168 ingredients. That's a lot of ingredients going into your body! Many of them could be causing more harm than good.

In the United States, no agency polices the skin care industry. Most people don't realize that the FDA does not oversee over-the-counter cosmetics like makeup, moisturizers, shampoos, and face and body washes. When doing my own research I often find that companies bend the truth when it comes to what exactly is in their skin care products. With skin care products, vague labels like "all natural" and "green" and even "organic" have been used and abused to the point that they are nearly meaningless. Look at all of the products on the market with images of green veggies or fresh fruits on the label—most will have an ingredients list filled with chemicals. It's all marketing—used to get your attention and your dollars. Just about any skin care product can make empty claims of being healthy or green or natural—it's up to you to be vigilant about what goes on, and eventually into, your body! Make sure you're not spending your money on false claims and marketing buzzwords.

To decipher all the information, I asked skin care expert Phil Masiello to teach us how to be savvier about ingredients and labeling.

Phil started his career in the food industry and then moved to skin care. He worked in sales and marketing that focused on launching natural and organic products into the retail channels. This insider's knowledge of natural and organic foods helped him learn a tremendous amount about ingredients and labeling laws in the United States.

In moving into the world of beauty products, Phil found that even experts in the field could be easily fooled by the dizzying array of claims, promises, and keywords found on skin care products. Manufacturers were taking shortcuts and not always being truthful. Phil's research revealed that there are four building blocks of skin care products and cosmetics:

1. A moisturizer can be any natural ingredient that is good for the target area. For example, rather than using harsh acids around the eye, combine carrot seed essential oil and coconut oil. For the body Phil suggests a blend of olive oil, coconut oil, avocado oil, and tamanu oil.

2. An emulsifier helps to mix oil and water to keep a product stable. Look for plant-based lecithin, aloe, and soy—these are all extracts that are natural emulsifiers. Unfortunately, many products are made with cheap chemical emulsifiers such as borax and triethanolamine, which are harmful and irritating and should be avoided.

3. A preservative is needed when water is an ingredient. Oil-based moisturizers don't need preservatives because bacteria and fungus can't grow in them. A blend of honeysuckle, tea tree oil, and salts will perform the same preservative function as parabens. Although it takes trial and error to get the proportion of these ingredients right, once you have it, it will work wonders.

Ask Carol

What are parabens and why do I need to worry about them?

ANSWER:

Paraben is a shorthand term that refers to chemical compounds of parahydroxybenzoic acid. They are used as preservatives to fight the growth of bacteria and fungus and can be found in shampoos, conditioners, moisturizers, deodorants, shaving gels, tanning lotions, sunscreen, personal lubricants, and toothpaste. Nearly all of the parabens used as preservatives are manmade and do not occur naturally. (Naturally occurring parabens have been found in blueberries, of all places!) Parabens can mimic the hormone estrogen and have been linked to breast cancer and reproductive issues.

Here are some paraben-free brands that can be found at your local drugstore or online:

- Bee Yummy
- The Body Deli
- Zum Soap Bars
- Age reversal technology by TotalMedicalAccess.com
- Board and Batten
- Uma Oils

If you want to know if your favorite skin care brand uses safe ingredients, check out the product safety guide compiled in the EWG's Skin Deep Cosmetics Database: www.ewg.org/skindeep.

4. Added *scents* make products smell amazing. Look for the term "essentials oils" on labels instead of the vague word "fragrance." Fragrances often just hide bad, unwanted ingredients, but essential oils are extracted from the skin of fruits like oranges, limes, and lemons, and from flowers and other parts of plants. Here is an interesting fact for you: bananas have no essential oil, so don't be fooled by a product that contains "natural banana fragrance." That "all natural" banana-scented hand soap was made in a lab!

As for labeling, Phil explained that there are just too many loopholes in the laws that don't favor the consumer at all. The FDA requires labeling standards if items follow a specific INCI (International Nomenclature of Cosmetic Ingredients) naming system—a system that uses names for ingredients based on the scientific or Latin name. INCI names often differ greatly from more common (consumer-known) names. To make things even more confusing, some words do have the same INCI name as the consumer-known one, such as lecithin (which is a natural emulsifying agent and one of the most important components of cells), but you still won't know whether the version used in a product comes from an animal or a plant, or whether it was extracted by chemical or mechanical means. There just isn't enough transparency in product labeling!

The Ten Worst Skin Care Ingredients

The labels on skin care and makeup products can be hard to understand. It's important you know what you are putting on your skin, though! To help, Phil and I compiled a list of what we think are the ten worst skin care ingredients so you will know what to avoid:

1. **Methyl, propyl, butyl, and ethyl parabens.** Widely used as preservatives to prevent bacterial and fungal growth in products. They are known to cause many allergic reactions, skin rashes, and more serious side effects like tumor growth and infertility.

   Healthy alternatives: Japanese honeysuckle and tea tree oil

2. **DMDM hydantoin and urea (imidazolidinyl).** These are also used as preservatives (similar to parabens). They are well established as a primary cause of contact dermatitis.

   Healthy alternatives: Japanese honeysuckle and tea tree oil

3. **Petrolatum.** This tends to interfere with the body's own natural moisturizing mechanism, leading to dry skin and chapping. If you purchase a product with petrolatum, you are being sold something that creates the very conditions it claims to alleviate. Manufacturers use petrolatum because it is an unbelievably cheap ingredient.

   Healthy alternatives: natural oils, such as tamanu oil, coconut oil, olive oil, palm oil, and avocado oil

4. **Propylene glycol.** This ingredient used in antifreeze is also used in makeup, toothpaste, and deodorant. It has been known to cause allergic reactions and even brain, liver, and kidney abnormalities. The U.S. Environmental Protection

Agency (EPA) requires workers to wear protective gloves, clothing, and goggles when working with propylene glycol. Is this something you want to put directly on your skin? Avoid it!

5. **PVP/VA copolymer.** A petroleum-derived chemical used in hairsprays, wave sets, and other cosmetics, this can be considered toxic, since particles may contribute to foreign bodies in the lungs of sensitive persons. Copolymer is an anti-aging and whitening agent; look for it on ingredients lists and avoid it.

6. **Sodium lauryl sulfate.** This synthetic substance is known for its detergent and foam-building abilities. An ingredient in the harsh cleansers used to clean car engines, garage floors, and vehicles at car washes, somehow it's still a popular ingredient in personal care products, including makeup, shampoo and conditioner, and toothpaste. Exposure to it can cause eye irritations, skin rashes, hair loss, scalp scurf (similar to dandruff), and other allergic reactions.

7. **Stearalkonium chloride.** A chemical used in hair conditioners and creams, it was developed by the fabric industry as a fabric softener.

8. **Synthetic colors.** They will be labeled as FD&C or D&C, followed by a color and a number, for example, FD&C Red No. 6 and D&C Green No. 6. Synthetic colors are believed to be cancer-causing agents. If a cosmetic contains them, don't use it. FD&C Red No. 4 is no longer available for use in foods because of a known threat to the adrenal glands and bladder.

Healthy alternatives: fruit extracts

9. **Synthetic fragrances.** The synthetic fragrances used in cosmetics can have as many as two hundred ingredients. There is no way to know what the chemicals are, since the label will simply list "fragrance." Some of the problems caused by these chemicals are headaches, dizziness, rash, hyperpigmentation, violent coughing, vomiting, and skin irritation; and they are even known to affect the central nervous system. Make sure your cosmetics get their scent from essential oils and not chemical "fragrances."

10. **Triethanolamine (TEA).** It's often used in cosmetics and in cement to adjust the pH. Yes, that's right—cosmetics and cement. It's used with fatty acids to convert acid to salt (stearate), which then becomes the base for a cleanser. TEA causes allergic reactions including eye problems and dryness of hair and skin, and can be toxic if absorbed into the body over a long period of time. It has also been linked to liver and kidney cancer.

Is it worth using products that contain these ingredients with the risks involved? Don't just buy what you see in advertisements; do your own research. You will be blown away by what popular brands get away with using in their products.

Brands That Care

To start you on the road toward purchasing healthier beauty products, I put together a list of some of my favorite brands. I've found that these products contain ingredients that help nourish your skin without allowing harmful chemicals in. Most of these products are made with real ingredients and you can actually eat them if you want (although I don't really advise this, as they might not always taste so good!).

MAKEUP

One of my favorite makeup brands is RMS Beauty. This line was created by New York City–based makeup artist Rose-Marie Swift. I've searched long and hard for healthy makeup, and RMS is the first makeup of its kind to really live up to the word "organic." I hope their success inspires other brands to follow their lead.

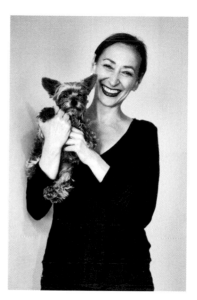

"Chemicals are redefining what beauty is in today's cosmetic industry, and that is not acceptable." —*Rose-Marie Swift,* founder of RMS Beauty

RMS's products are 100 percent free of harmful chemicals and also work to nourish your skin with healthy and beautifying results. They are filled with high-quality raw ingredients (my favorite!). Rose-Marie explains: "When a raw material is processed for use in cosmetics, it typically undergoes a lengthy process. I discovered the majority of ingredients used for natural cosmetics (organic or not) go through multiple steps from deodorizing, refining, and fractionating during production, to heating to extremely high temperatures again during manufacturing. These processes render the "natural" ingredients equivalent to man-made chemicals, stripping away all beneficial nutrients and enzymes that support healthy skin and life."

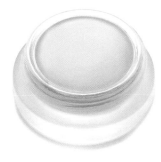

RMS Beauty products, on the other hand, are formulated with raw, food-grade, organic ingredients in their natural state, from cultivation straight through to manufacturing. Organic, raw ingredients like cocoa and shea butters, and cold-pressed organic jojoba oil are similar to the naturally occurring oils in human skin and contain some of the most powerful, nourishing, and healing qualities it thirsts for.

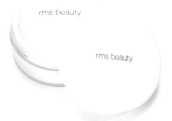

RMS Beauty also takes extreme care to use minimal heat in the manufacturing process, thus preserving every vital nutrient that nature provides. Unlike today's synthetic counterparts, this technique allows natural healing and life force attributes—such as enzymes, minerals, vitamins, and, most important, antioxidants—to remain fully intact and naturally penetrate and rejuvenate skin. For gorgeous, modern color, Rose-Marie chooses tints from pure, raw, uncorrupted, and uncoated minerals.

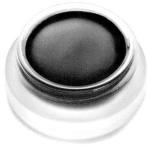

The results? A color makeup line designed to work synergistically with the skin, rather than just covering it up! When you apply the products, their natural life-giving nutrients interact with your skin to promote hydration, softness, radiance, and instant vitality.

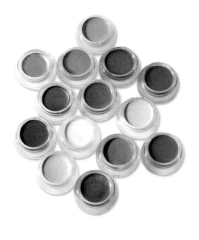

Carol's Tip

My favorite RMS products are their "Sacred" color lip gloss, which is an amazing shade of red with a hint of pink, and their Living Luminizer, which helps make your eyes and cheekbones glow. You can purchase them online at www.rmsbeauty.com.

DEODORANT

It's not just skin creams that have harmful ingredients. Deodorants can be just as bad—especially since you scrape your skin by shaving and then put them directly near your lymph nodes. I had Jaime Schmidt, owner of Schmidt's Deodorant, on *A Healthy You & Carol Alt* to discuss the harmful chemicals lurking in deodorants. What I love about Jaime's product is that instead of being in the typical stick or roll-on form that most people are used to, this paste deodorant is applied directly to your armpit skin with your fingers.

First you warm the deodorant in your hands and then you rub it into your armpits like a lotion.

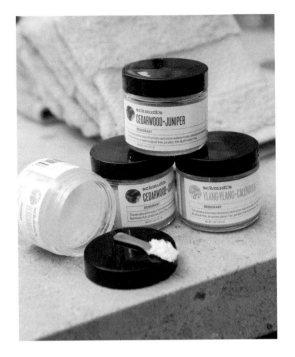

Some people might find the experience a little weird, and I agree that it takes a little getting used to, but when did armpits become a gross thing? They are a part of our bodies just like everything else. Jaime explained that this rubbing of the armpit actually helps drain the lymphatic system, which is often a spot where women in particular get cancer.

The consumer market is full of endless deodorant options, so I had Jaime explain how to make better choices when choosing a deodorant to wear every day.

Which ingredients should be avoided, and what are the safer alternatives?

- Aluminum is the active ingredient in most antiperspirants. It works by blocking the sweat glands to keep sweat from getting to the skin's surface. Some research has shown that daily use of aluminum-based antiperspirants may increase the risk of developing diseases such as Alzheimer's and cancer. Schmidt's Deodorant uses arrowroot powder to absorb moisture while allowing for the body's natural process of perspiring.

- Triclosan is another common ingredient found in commercial deodorants. It has antibacterial properties and is the odor-killing ingredient in antiperspirants.

Triclosan is classified as a pesticide by the U.S. Food and Drug Administration and as a probable carcinogen by the Environmental Protection Agency. A safer way to prevent the growth of odor-causing bacteria is to use baking soda and extracts of the hops plant.

- Parabens are synthetic preservatives. They are estrogen mimicking, and possible side effects of constant exposure to them include early puberty in children, organ toxicity, and an increased risk of hormonal cancers. Schmidt's Deodorant uses a gluten-free, soy-based form of vitamin E as a preservative instead.

- Phthalates are chemical stabilizers that help the product cling to the skin. These hormone disruptors have been linked to a variety of health issues, including higher risk of birth defects. A safer alternative is cocoa butter, which is also high in antioxidants and rich in minerals.

- Propylene glycol is a petroleum-based material that gives deodorant a slick consistency, making the product easier to apply to the skin. Studies have shown that in large quantities it can cause damage to the central nervous system, liver, and heart. Natural shea butter, which moisturizes and protects delicate underarm skin, can be used in the place of this dangerous additive.

- Synthetic fragrance oils are used in the majority of conventional deodorant brands. Potential side effects range from skin irritation and chronic headaches to fatigue and endocrine imbalances. Schmidt's Deodorant has found a safer approach to adding fragrance, using pure essential oils extracted from plant material. Essential oils offer antibacterial, antioxidant, deodorizing, and healing properties.

- Deodorant is a fundamental part of our daily hygiene routine, but not always something we give much thought to. Check your deodorant (yes—right now, while you are reading this!). Make sure your deodorant doesn't contain any of these ingredients and if it does—throw it out and try a safer alternative. Now, I'll be here when you're back!

Carol's Tip

I also like to just powder my armpits with baking soda. I know of nothing that works better to absorb odor!

ORAL CARE

As we discussed earlier, it's important to be conscious of what ingredients are in your toothpaste and mouthwash. Even knowing what your toothbrush is made of is a smart idea. All of these ingredients are absorbed into your body—so they matter! One of my favorite companies for dental health is Living Libations. Nadine Artemis is the co-creator of Living Libations, an amazing line of serums, elixirs, and essential oils for those seeking the purest of the pure.

Nadine suggests: "Before you do anything else, ditch the toxic synthetic and chemical toothpastes, whiteners, and mouthwashes that clutter your bathroom counter. Many of these products come loaded with lauryl sulfates and therefore have the warning label 'May be harmful if swallowed,' so do you really want to put them in your mouth?"

The chemicals in most oral care products, including many of the brands sold in health-food stores, use ingredients that are more appropriate for industrial purposes than for cleaning the delicate tissue of the mouth. Stop using them!

Nature provides beautiful and effective botanicals that attend to our health and beauty and work wonders on our teeth. Essential oils distilled from organically grown, aromatic plants potently clean and protect our oral ecology and can actually boost our overall health.

Here are some of my favorite products from Living Libations:

Healthy Gums Clay Toothpaste: It contains infusions of rose, peppermint, clove, oregano, cinnamon, sea buckthorn, tea tree, and thyme; pyrophyllite clay; zeolite; coconut oil; saponified olive oil; and sodium bicarbonate. Pyrophyllite clay is a powerful alchemical agent that promotes the transformation and transmission of electromagnetic energy. Clay absorbs toxins in the mouth, including heavy metals, viruses, bacteria, and parasites. The rich silica and mineral content of the clay nourishes both teeth and gums, improving the overall health of the entire mouth.

Healthy Gum Drops: If you don't like flossing, you will love Healthy Gum Drops! They contain supercritical extracts and essences of sea buckthorn berry, oregano, peppermint, clove, tea tree, cinnamon, and thyme linalool. These organic and wild-crafted ingredients create an effective antibacterial, antifungal ointment for all aspects of oral care. Add one drop to your toothbrush, or glide a drop over dental floss to cleanse the tiny spaces in between the teeth.

Do It Yourself!

A lot of people, including myself, like to make their own DIY hair and skin care products. This way you can know exactly what's in the products you are using. And as an added bonus, making your own products can also save you money! I've put together some of my favorite DIY at-home treatments and products for you. Most of these recipes take less than five minutes to make and you can find all the ingredients in your kitchen or local health-food store.

Don't be scared or overwhelmed to give DIY a go—try it out! Have fun with it! You never know, maybe it will inspire you to create your own body care line one day.

HYDRATING FACE MASKS

—By Carmindy, makeup artist and creator
of Carmindy & Co.

For dry or combination skin:

¼ cup yogurt
1 medium banana
2 tablespoons honey

Blend all the ingredients together (into a paste). Spread on the skin and leave on for 20 minutes.

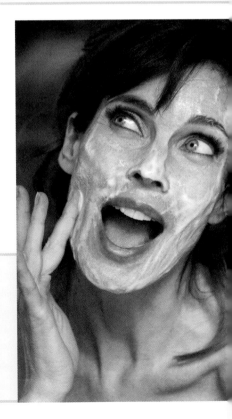

Carol's Tip

Honey has antibacterial and anti-inflammatory properties, and even rejuvenates skin cells.

For oily or acne-prone skin:

½ cucumber

2 tablespoons rolled oats

½ lemon

1 tablespoon honey

Blend all the ingredients together. Spread on the skin and leave on for 20 minutes.

Carol's Tip

Cucumber is a natural astringent.

NATURAL FACE SCRUB

—By Carmindy, makeup artist and creator of Carmindy & Co.

A simple (but effective!) brown sugar scrub. Brown sugar naturally exfoliates, and many people don't realize that those microbeads in commercial scrubs are actually plastic.

½ cup honey

2 tablespoons rolled oats

½ cup packed brown
  sugar

1 tablespoon coconut oil

1 drop of essential oil of
  your choice

Blend all the ingredients together. Apply to the face, neck, and chest and use daily.

DIY NATURAL TOOTHPASTE

—By Nadine Artemis, Living Libations

This toothpaste foams to lift up bacteria and heal the gums. The essential oils have antibacterial and antifungal properties.

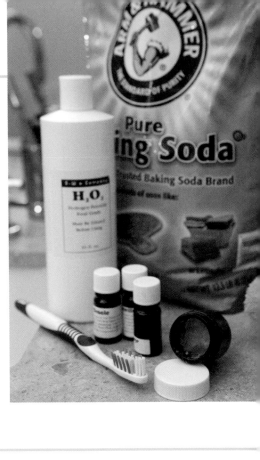

1 teaspoon baking soda

1 teaspoon apple cider vinegar

1 drop of essential oil such as clove, cinnamon, neem, or peppermint

Blend all the ingredients together and use daily.

DIY FOAMING HAND SOAP

—By Katie the "Wellness Mama," www.wellnessmama.com

This is an incredibly simple, natural, and frugal foaming hand soap that cleans without chemicals or antibacterial agents. Use it as you would any regular foaming soap. The best water to use is distilled or boiled, unless the soap will be used within a few weeks. Be sure to add the castile soap to the water, not the other way around, to avoid creating too many bubbles.

Water

About 2 tablespoons liquid castile soap

½ teaspoon liquid oil, like olive or almond (optional)

A few drops of essential oils of your choice for scent (optional)

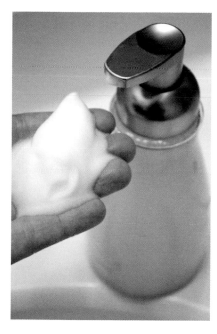

1. Fill a foaming soap dispenser with water to within 1 inch of the top (leaving room for the bulky foaming pump and the soap to be added).

2. Add the castile soap to the dispenser.

3. Add the oil (not necessary, but it helps preserve the life of the dispenser) and any essential oils if you are using them.

4. Insert the pump and close tightly. Lightly swish the dispenser to mix the soap.

DIY DRY SHAMPOO FOR DARK OR LIGHT HAIR

—*By Katie the "Wellness Mama," www.wellnessmama.com*

Dry shampoo is all the rage now! Be careful, as commercially available products can be filled with chemicals. Wellness Mama's dry shampoo is naturally scented with essential oils and can be customized to your hair type. You can apply it with an old makeup brush or just with your hands!

Light Hair

¼ cup arrowroot powder or non-GMO cornstarch
5 drops of essential oil of your choice (optional)

Dark Hair

2 tablespoons arrowroot or cornstarch
2 tablespoons unsweetened cocoa powder
5 drops of essential oil of your choice (optional)

Put the arrowroot (and cocoa powder, if making the dark hair version) in a bowl. Add the essential oil, if using, and mix with a spoon. Store the shampoo in a small jar or old powder container.

To use, apply to the roots or oily parts of your hair. Comb the powder through your hair and style as usual.

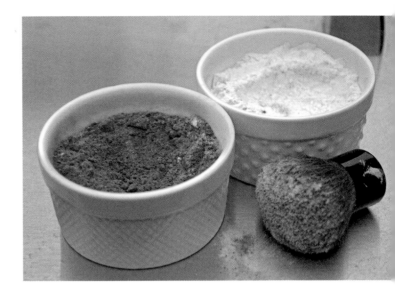

ONLINE DIY RESOURCES

There are many amazing DIY health bloggers these days! You can check out more great DIYs from Katie the "Wellness Mama," www.wellnessmama .com. You can also visit A Delightful Home, www.adelightfulhome.com, and Hello Natural, http://HelloNatural.co.

Your Mouth and Your Health

It's been ingrained in our heads to brush our teeth since we were young. We've always known this was important, but recent research has revealed that the benefits of brushing go beyond having a great smile or pleasant breath. Most of us don't realize how much our oral health impacts the entire body! Yes, entire body! The health of your gums and teeth can give your dentist a good indication of whether you may develop heart disease or diabetes in the future.

You know a topic is important when I dedicate an entire episode of *A Healthy You & Carol Alt* to it! Cancer and nutrition expert Dr. Nicholas Gonzalez explained, "Important clues to your overall health lie in your teeth, gums, and even tongue. Alternatively, mouth problems can also cause problems in other parts of the body. Different parts of our mouth are connected to different organs in our body."

Did you know that billions (yes, billions!) of bacteria and other microscopic critters live in the mouth? Though some of these bacteria are good, a lot are bad and can cause harm throughout your body. If you don't practice good oral health care, the bad bacteria can grow out of control and move through the circulatory system.

According to Reid Winick, DDS, founder of Dentistry for Health in New York City, research has also shown a link between oral health and heart disease, heart attack, stroke, and diabetes. It's important to care for your teeth to prevent cavities, and also to avoid root canals or tooth extractions. These procedures, according to Dr. Winick, "can change your bite, often leading to issues like TMJ. If the bite is off by even one millimeter, your whole skull can be off. TMJ is a central part of the skull and, when it moves, so do the skull bones, resulting in headaches, reduced cognitive ability, decreased memory, and worse."

Another oral health issue to consider is the use of mercury fillings. If you've had cavities filled I suggest you keep reading. Dr. Veselin Shumantov, dentist with the Center for Advanced Dentistry, elaborated on the dangers of fillings: "Silver fillings (mercury) have been around since the 1950s and were hailed because of their strength. Mercury is one of the most toxic heavy metals, though, because it can cross the blood and brain barrier. It is responsible for headaches, tremors, weakness, and more. Some people who have had mercury fillings have been diagnosed with MS symptoms."

Now that we are aware of the problems lurking in the mouth, how can we prevent them? I turned to Nadine Artemis, author of *Holistic Dental Care* and owner of Living Libations, and again to Dr. Winick for advice:

Artemis:

- **Make your own toothpaste** (see the recipe on page 188).

- **Help your teeth remineralize through your diet** by adding fat-soluble vitamins and minerals (such as vitamins D_3, K_2, and A) and eliminating or treating things that might be making the saliva acidic, such as your toothpaste, grains in your diet, or having acidic blood.

Winick:

- **Use a Hydro Floss oral irrigator.** When it comes to removing bacteria from under your gums, flossing is subpar at best. Instead, a Hydro Floss actually gives your gums a daily shower and helps wash the pathogenic, bad bacteria away.

- **Stop drinking soda.** It's well known that sugar causes cavities and plaque. But what might not be as obvious is that no matter how thoroughly one brushes, it is difficult to remove all sweeteners from the teeth. This is because most sugary foods and drinks contain corn syrup—a sweetener that coats the teeth and hides in cracks and crevices, where it festers and decays your teeth.

- **Maintain a balanced pH.** A low pH in your mouth means it's an acidic environment, which is a breeding ground for unwanted bacteria. This level of pH leaves you more susceptible to cavities and gum disease. Keep your pH at an optimal level by eating a diet rich in whole foods, including plenty of fruits and vegetables.

Ask Carol

Does oil pulling really work? Or is it just a passing fad?

ANSWER:

Oil pulling seems to be all the rage lately. I've been oil pulling for years with my boyfriend, Alexei, and I can testify that it really works. My gums are strong and my teeth are whiter than ever. I asked Dr. Gonzalez what he thinks of oil pulling. He mentioned that it isn't a new technique. It is something that has been practiced by Ayurvedic physicians for a couple thousand years. Ayurvedic doctors, he said, are very smart—and they knew that many health problems begin in the mouth.

For those of you who haven't heard of it, oil pulling is a technique where you put a tablespoon of oil (Dr. Gonzalez recommends sesame or coconut oil) in your mouth and swish it around for 15 minutes. As you swish, bacteria and toxins are drawn out of the body—they get "stuck" in the oil—and when you spit it out, they are removed.

It's pretty simple and doesn't take that much time. Try it! I suggest doing it first thing in the morning but it's up to you. Just make sure you brush well, teeth and tongue, immediately after.

Healthy Hair

Whether she's rocking a short pixie cut or a long and shiny mane, a woman's hair can make her feel confident and sexy. A hairstyle can exude femininity or rebellion and often completes a woman's signature look. By far, the question I get asked the most is "What is your hair secret?" My secret? You can probably guess by now: a healthy diet with a sprinkle of good genes.

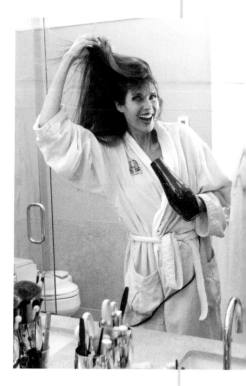

Your hair is 91 percent protein and is made up of long chains of amino acids. It's important to eat a diet full of fatty acids, which are raw fats, and essential amino acids, which are raw proteins, to keep your hair healthy and strong. They are the building blocks that your body uses to build and restore itself. Unfortunately, your hair and nails are the last to receive these nutrients and often get neglected. It's important to eat enough fatty acids and essential amino acids so that there is enough for every part of your body.

Carol's Tip

Some great hair foods are:

- Carpaccio (raw meats and fish)
- Dark leafy vegetables
- Essential fatty acids, including those found in raw milk cheese, raw butter, Udo's Choice oils, olive oil, coconut oil, and fatty fish like salmon. Remember, raw dairy is *not* the same as pasteurized (which means cooked).

HAIR AND AGING

As you get older, you'll start to see signs of aging in your hair. The color might fade to gray, the density decreases, and the texture often becomes brittle. Although you can't completely control this process, since some of it has to do with your genes, the food you eat and how you treat your hair does play a large part in keeping your hair looking youthful.

Gray hair can often start to sneak in as early as your midthirties. The color in your hair comes from the same place as the color in your skin: melanocytes, which produce melanin. Your hair cells produce little bits of hydrogen peroxide—yes, the chemical that makes hair blond—which is, in turn, broken down by the enzyme catalase. As we age, catalase production decreases and the hydrogen peroxide begins to block those pigment-producing melanocytes, making for less colored, or gray, strands.

I think aging gracefully is wonderful and beautiful, but, like you, I still want to push aging off as long as possible. Besides eating healthy, there are some tricks of the trade to help you age as naturally as possible but keep a youthful look and glow.

COLORING YOUR HAIR

If you are going to color your hair, Marco Pelusi, owner of Marco Pelusi Salon in LA, recommends going with a nontoxic dye. Marco also explained that as women age they lose pigment in both their skin and hair. As a result, many women can easily look washed out, "especially if the woman has too much gray,

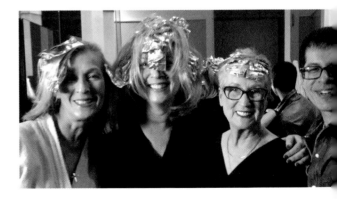

My sisters and my mom having fun with Marco Pelusi of the Marco Pelusi Salon. *Left to right:* Karen; Chris; my mom, Muriel; and Marco.

too many highlights or ash tones"—and that can appear to put as many as ten years on a person's face. Many people settle on a hair color in their twenties and then stick with that through life. Marco suggests making sure you update your hair and its color every few years to complement your changing looks.

LOSS OF DENSITY

As you age, your hair also loses its density. All women will experience some level of hair loss as they get older. In most cases, the loss will be minor, but some women may find they can see their scalps easily through their hair, particularly at the perimeter areas.

One common cause of hair loss is low thyroid function, which occurs commonly in women experiencing menopause. The fluctuations in hormone levels of women during menopause can also cause hair loss, as can the emotional and physical stress that many women feel as they get older.

As we age, the growth rate of the hair slows down, meaning that when hairs are shed, they are replaced more slowly. If you feel that your hair loss is somehow atypical, talk to your doctor about it.

Carol's Tip

Want fuller, more luxurious hair? Try my rosemary oil hair mask! I make this mask at home to keep my hair looking shiny and vibrant. Mix together 1 egg, ½ avocado, ¼ cup coconut oil, and 15 drops of rosemary oil. Put the mixture on your hair and leave it for 20 minutes. Rinse with cool water.

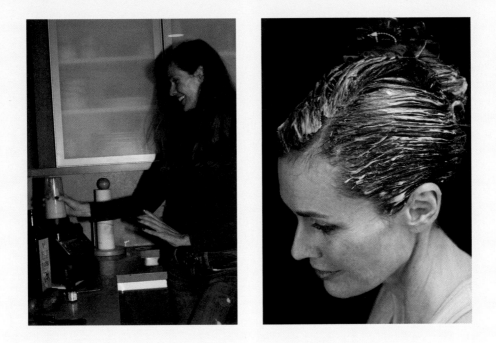

CHANGE IN TEXTURE

After a certain age, many women notice that their hair becomes drier, and the texture often seems coarse and brittle. This is because the body's production of sebum, a naturally created lubricant of the skin and hair, slows down as you age. Sebum production decreases by 10 percent every ten years.

You can help this process by eating a healthy diet rich in antioxidants and vitamins A, E, and C, as well as omega-3 fatty acids.

My hairdresser, Tatiana Boyko, suggests castor oil to help make hair more silky. Rub it into your roots with a drop of eucalyptus oil (which helps stimulate your scalp) and work it down the hair shaft to the ends, then sleep with your hair in a shower cap overnight. Your hair should be shining and strong in no time!

Carol's Tip

Silica, which is found in cucumbers, cabbage, and celery, improves the elasticity of hair, preventing split ends! I also like silica-rich horsetail tea. One word of warning about horsetail tea: it has a bit of caffeine in it, so don't drink too much at once to try to load up on silica! Doesn't work that way!

BALDNESS

Baldness seems to be a growing problem for both men and women, and until recently, there have been very limited options for growing your hair back naturally. I had hair specialist Elaine Magliacano, owner of Anagen Hair Solutions, explain a new technology that her company has to grow hair. They use cosmetic lasers, which help bring blood to the hair follicles—it's that increased blood flow that promotes growth.

This laser technique has an 85 percent success rate, and there are no harmful side effects. The catch? The process takes about eight months to a year and the client must come in twice a week for 20- to 30-minute sessions. That might seem like a lot of time, but for some the results are well worth it.

Ask Carol

What shampoo and conditioner do you use on your hair? It's so silky and long!

ANSWER:

My first step was to take the harsh minerals out of my bathing water. I installed a water filter in my shower, and this step alone changed the texture of my hair. Second, I'm a big fan of pH Miracle Young Phorever shampoo and conditioner. You can buy it online at www .phmiracleliving.com.

I also like Soignée Botanical Shampoo, which you can buy online at www.soignee.com.

What Are Your Nails Telling You?

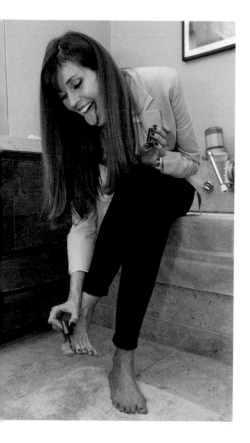

Your nails may be a good indication of your personal grooming habits and are often used as accessories for fashion, but they can also give you clues about your overall health. Our bodies are quite smart, and if we are properly in tune with them, they often let us know when something is not right. The problem is that many of us are going through life too fast and we fail to notice these small subtleties.

Right now—take a second to look at your nails (take that polish off!). Do you see anything abnormal? Your nails should be smooth and have a light half circle where the nail starts to grow. Notice anything different? You might have a white spot here and there, or perhaps some discoloration. This might not look like much to you, but to a trained eye it does. I spoke with Dr. Robert L. Bard, founder of the Bard Cancer Center, who explained to me that your nails hold valuable clues to your body's overall health. Nail problems may reflect a medical disorder or a local change in the underlying bone and adjacent blood vessels.

Dr. Bard pointed out some nail deformities to watch out for, as they are linked to disease:

- Nail clubbing (the nail points down, looking like the round part of an upside-down spoon) can signal pulmonary problems and can indicate iron deficiency or anemia.

- Vertical lines can point to arthritis or injury.

- Horizontal lines, called Beau's lines, can be a sign of diabetes, circulatory disease, past high fever, or malnutrition.

- Brittle nails can indicate thyroid malfunction or a parathyroid benign tumor (parathyroid adenoma), which if caught early is curable.

- Rippled nails may be an early sign of psoriasis or inflammatory arthritis.

- Yellow nails can indicate a fungal infection. In rare cases, yellow nails can signal a more serious condition, such as thyroid disease, lung disease, diabetes, or psoriasis.

- A bluish tint to your nails may indicate that your body is not getting enough oxygen. This could indicate a lung problem, such as emphysema, or even a heart problem.

- Pale nails can be a sign of serious illness, such as anemia, congestive heart failure, liver disease, or malnutrition.

- White nails can indicate liver problems, such as hepatitis.

- Nails that are opaque but show a dark band beneath the top of the nail are called Terry's nails. This can be a sign of several conditions, including congestive heart failure, diabetes, liver disease, and malnutrition. It can also be a sign of aging.

- Localized bone irregularities or overgrowth might loosen the nail plate, allowing for splitting and fungus infection.

Know every part of your body! Be conscious of a change in your nails. If you notice changes or abnormalities in your fingernails, don't dismiss them. Make an appointment with your doctor. Prevention is always key!

HEALTH HAZARDS LURKING IN NAIL SALONS

Who doesn't love going to the nail salon for a relaxing mani-pedi? It's one of the few places I can retreat to soak away stress. But could those warm towels and tools be doing more harm than good? How do you know what's safe and what's not? Also, what ingredients are in that nail polish?

I spoke with Dr. Karin Hehenberger, the founder of Lyfebulb, a platform for people living with chronic disease, to get to the bottom of this. Dr. Hehenberger says you can continue to enjoy going to the nail salon, but you need to make sure you take some precautions. She suggests checking up on the salon before you go. While you can tell a lot just looking inside a salon, it's important to also check out reviews, too. During a pedicure, don't let the nail technician scrub or scrape the bottoms of your feet too much, as this can cause open wounds that can lead to infections. If you are already in a salon, Dr. Hehenberger suggests getting a manicure first, as this will allow you to watch firsthand if the technicians properly clean their tools. It is best when salons use an autoclave, which is a machine used in medical environments that produces steam and pressure for disinfecting equipment.

Ask Carol

Do you recommend any brand of nail polish?

ANSWER:

I look for nail polishes that do not have these top five questionable ingredients:

- Formaldehyde (to make nails harder)

- Dibutyl phthalate

- Toluene

- Formaldehyde resin (to strengthen nails)

- Camphor (even though it occurs naturally, camphor is *not* nontoxic)

I look for the following brands:

- Nature Dry aka Dazzle Dry

- Priti

- Vapour Organic Beauty

- RGB

- Scotch Naturals

- Tenoverten

- Kure Bazaar

- Acquarella

- Chanel

- NCLA

- Spa Ritual

- Mineral Fusion

Remember—what you eat is at the forefront of every one of my beauty and skin care tips! A healthy, nutritious diet filled with vegetables and unprocessed food is your foundation on which to build. Diet plus exercising and caring about what you are putting on your body are all part of showing your body self-love and, I promise, will make every part of your life better. Be conscious of the ingredients in your makeup and skin and hair care products. Your skin is absorbing everything you apply. Read labels carefully and always opt for a natural solution or ingredients. Doing so will make a difference in the long run.

Your beauty comes from the inside first. Remember that every time you look in the mirror, and hold your head up high!

PART 4

Aging

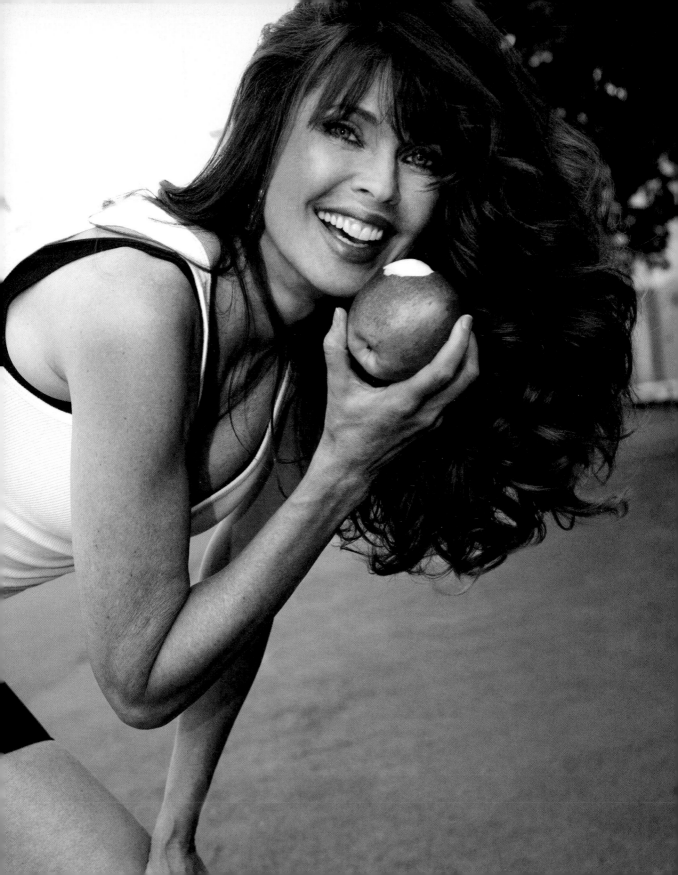

Y ou'll notice that I have already touched upon the subject of aging as it relates to diet, fitness, and beauty, but I thought it would be a good idea to include an entire section about this topic, since, well, it happens to every one of us every day!

Many people are constantly looking for the next miracle cream or treatment that's going to make them look twenty-five again, but sadly, it doesn't exist. Anti-aging products and cosmetics are one of the biggest commodities in the United States, generating about fifty billion dollars a year. But I've said it once, and I'm saying it again: the keys to aging well are (drumroll, please!) diet and exercise. But don't just take my word for it—let's investigate.

When you work in the beauty industry as I have, and especially in front of the camera, you are confronted with the harsh realities of aging on a daily basis. There is always a younger face right around the corner, and this fosters inevitable insecurities within you. Obviously there is no way to stop Father Time from ticking away, and there is no way to stop your face or body from showing signs of aging (I'm sorry to inform you that that "miracle cream" you spent $70 on will not actually be a facelift in a bottle), but there are certainly steps you can take to age gracefully and to remain glowing and beautiful throughout your life.

We all hear the clichés about how fifty is the new thirty-five and sixty is the new fifty and so on. Well, I remember vividly when the compliments I received about my looks began to have qualifying accompaniments about my age. "You look great" became "You look great for your age." And I was not happy about that. It would be disingenuous if I did not admit to caring a lot about my physical appearance and devoting considerable attention to it. And through the years I have tried all kinds of potions and formulas that promised to keep me looking young. But since I changed to a raw diet, I have expanded this focus to include how I feel and think and act and move and sleep and what kind of energy I exude to those around me.

In short, aging gracefully has become a 360-degree lifestyle pursuit for me, with the intended goal being not only to look pretty but also, and more important, to feel like I am doing the best I can in every other category as well. Hopefully this will lead not only to more years of life but to more life in my years as well.

In this part, I want to explore how our bodies react to aging and what we can do physically, emotionally, and spiritually to put a positive spin on some of the best years of our lives—the years to come!

The Age Factor:
Identifying the Main Culprits

I often hear people complain that they have bad genes and there's nothing they can do to stop the ravages of aging. This just sounds like an excuse to me! As I mentioned, aging will happen—it's inevitable—but you can slow down this process with (you probably guessed it!) your diet and lifestyle. According to Jonny Bowden, nutritionist and author of *The Most Effective Ways to Live Longer,* only 15 to 20 percent of the aging process has to do with our genes. The rest has to do with how we treat our bodies, which determines whether, like a light switch, we turn the good genes on and the bad genes off. Everything we've discussed so far, or will discuss in this section of the book—what we eat and drink, if we exercise daily, proper sleep, finding a passion and purpose in life, learning to love ourselves, the harmful products in our beauty and household cleaning routines—plays a role in the aging process. These factors are the light switch. Knowing this should feel empowering, as you are the one in control of everything I just listed.

My whole life changed when I realized that I was the one who had the power. It affected the way I thought about everything. I was sick because I wasn't treating my body properly and giving it what it needed to flourish and repair itself. I'm very thankful I was introduced to raw food and that my life turned around the way it did, as it has allowed me to age gracefully. This change in my mind-set also helped me ignite my passion, which is teaching people how to make the change I did and become healthy and have more energy than ever. You can do it, too!

Here are some of the biggest factors that I've found that can affect the way your body handles aging:

- **Stress:** You've heard stress mentioned throughout the book. It's a biggie! If you want to live a long and happy life, you need to learn how to cope with stress. Stress impacts inflammation in your body, which is the cause of many chronic diseases. It's inevitable that we are going to have stressors in life—a presentation at work, getting your kids to school on time, or even taking out the garbage—but it's how we deal with them that matters. If the body is in constant fight-or-flight mode in reaction to stress, it will suffer. To better deal with the stressors in your life and maintain physical and emotional equilibrium, I suggest trying some of the following stress relievers: get some fresh air (nature does wonders!), meditate (Russell Simmons explains his meditation style on page 150), do yoga, get connected to your spiritual side, take a bath, express gratitude toward someone, or exercise. Realize what situations you are in control of and focus on changing them so they are not causes of stress in your life.

Jessica Ortner, author of *The Tapping Solution for Weight Loss & Body Confidence,* suggests another way to combat stress: a releasing technique called tapping. Tapping helps you work through stress and actually helps lower your production of cortisol, the hormone our bodies release when we're stressed. To tap, you gently press nine acupressure points on the body—beginning with the side of the hand, then moving to the eyebrow, side of the eye, under the eye, under the nose, the chin, the collarbone, under the armpit, and ending with the top of the head—as you repeat a "setup statement" that vocalizes your emotional and physical stress. (You can head to my blog, www.carolalt.com, for a demonstration!) Jessica states, "When you're feeling centered and strong, tapping allows you to get your power back."

- **An unhealthy diet:** Here we are again! I'm sure you have now realized the importance of the food you eat to the rest of your life. As we have discussed, a diet full of processed foods is hard for the body to properly digest and is filled with harmful ingredients that add up over time and can lead to inflammation, which causes disease. Your diet should consist of organic and unprocessed real foods—or raw ones.

- **Not getting the right amount of vitamin D:** Vitamin D is essential for bone health. Recent research also shows that it may have other benefits, such as fighting depression and colds. A lot of people shy away from sun exposure, but a little bit (about fifteen minutes a day) is good for you. Increasing your intake of vitamin D can have profound benefits for your health. In the summer, boost your vitamin D level for free by careful and safe sun exposure—our bodies synthesize vitamin D from sunlight. In the winter, I suggest taking vitamin D supplements. Very few foods contain vitamin D, but you can add fatty fish, such as salmon, trout, mackerel, or eel, to your diet to increase your intake of vitamin D.

- **Not eating antioxidant-rich foods:** Antioxidants have gained popularity in the past few years for a reason. Good sources of antioxidants include blueberries, cranberries, blackberries, raspberries, strawberries, cherries, beans, and artichokes.

  NOTE: When a food suddenly gets great press for its antioxidant content, many people load up on that one food. You need to realize that overeating that one food alone will not make your diet healthier. Antioxidants are found in a variety of foods, so eat a wide spectrum of foods to incorporate as many of them into your meals as you can.

- **Not using enough oil:** Coconut oil is a wonderful anti-aging food. It is known to reduce your risk of heart disease and lower your cholesterol, among many other health benefits. Besides ingesting it, I also put it all over my body as a lotion. Double whammy!

- **Not getting enough natural resveratrol:** Resveratrol is one of the front-runners in the anti-aging race. Although resveratrol is the antioxidant found in red wine, I can't recommend drinking wine in the hopes of extending your life because the alcohol in wine can harm your body's delicate hormonal balance. Instead, you can get resveratrol from other food sources, such as whole grape skins and seeds, raspberries, mulberries, and peanuts.

- **Not enough regular exercise:** As we have discussed, regular exercise benefits every part of your life. Studies show that engaging in regular moderate to vigorous exercise as you age can help prevent or delay the onset of hypertension, obesity, heart disease, osteoporosis, as well as help prevent falls that lead to hip fractures. It's best to exercise at all ages of your life, and it's never too late to start! It's been shown that even individuals who start exercising in their seventies can substantially increase both their strength and endurance.

- **Overexposure to chemicals, toxins, and pollutants in your home:** Conventional cleaning products are known to be among the most toxic products found in your home. Many contain carcinogens or suspected carcinogens. This includes household cleaners, soaps, personal hygiene products, air fresheners, bug sprays, lawn pesticides, and insecticides, just to name a few.

The Environmental Working Group recently conducted a study of household cleaners and published the results in its Cleaners Database Hall of Shame (you can find it online at www.ewg.org/cleaners/hallofshame). The EWG found that 53 percent of regular household cleaning products contained lung-harming ingredients. Here is the EWG's list of some of the common chemicals found in household products that you should be aware of:

* Chlorine bleach (sodium hypochlorite): If mixed with ammonia, vinegar, or other acid-based cleaners, bleach will release toxic chloramine gas; short-term exposure to this gas can cause mild asthmatic symptoms or more serious respiratory problems. Never mix bleach with these other substances.

* Petroleum distillates: Found in metal polishes, these chemicals can irritate the eyes and lungs; longer-term exposure can damage the nervous system, kidneys, eyes, and skin.

* Ammonia: Can irritate eyes and lungs and cause headaches.

* Phenol and cresol: Found in disinfectants, these chemicals can cause diarrhea, fainting, dizziness, and kidney and liver damage if ingested.

* Nitrobenzene: Found in furniture and floor polishes. If inhaled it can cause shallow breathing, and if ingested it can cause poisoning and death. This substance has also been linked to cancer and birth defects.

* Formaldehyde: Used as a preservative in many household products, formaldehyde is a suspected human carcinogen that can irritate your eyes, throat, skin, and lungs.

* Naphthalene: Found in mothballs, this suspected carcinogen may damage the eyes, blood cells, liver, kidneys, skin, and central nervous system.

* Hydrochloric acid or sodium acid sulfate: Found in toilet bowl cleaners, these chemicals can burn the skin and cause blindness if splashed in the eyes or can burn the stomach if ingested.

It's also a great idea to use nontoxic food ingredients for cleaning—this is sure to be the natural way! Head over to my blog (www.carolalt.com) for tips on how to use baking soda, lemons, and vinegar to clean your house.

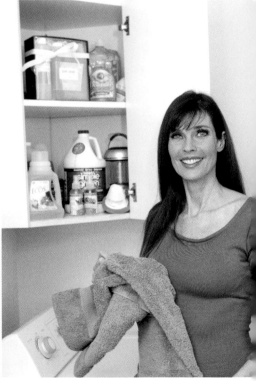

Taking the time to replace the products you use every day with nontoxic or natural alternatives will help your overall health.

Carol's Tip

I've done a lot of research on nontoxic household products! My favorite eco-friendly cleaners are made by companies such as Eco-Me and Earth Friendly Products. The list of green cleaners has tripled in the past five years! It's great to see that so many brands with quality and nonharmful ingredients are appearing on the market.

- **Exposure to EMFs:** EMFs (electromagnetic fields) are all around you these days and it's impossible to completely avoid them; they're produced by your wireless Internet connection, keyboard, and mouse; your cell phone; power lines; and electrical wires.

  Research shows there might be a connection between EMFs and aging. I spoke with Camilla Rees, founder of ElectromagneticHealth.org and a campaigner for radiation-free schools, to get her advice on how to be. She suggests:

  1. Use hard-wired telephone connections at home. Minimize cell phone use at every opportunity to lower total daily, and cumulative, radiofrequency exposure.

  2. Cell phones should not be near the body, daytime or nighttime. Keep them out of your pockets!

  3. Strive to make your bedroom as electromagnetically clean as possible: no cell phones, portable phones, or wireless routers or other computer equipment.

4. Use caution with computer monitors. Be aware that many new computer screens, including those of desktops, laptops, tablets, and even smartphones, use glossy, backlit LED screens that can cause eye strain and headaches. Seek out the older matte LCD screens whenever possible to minimize eye and brain dysfunction.

5. Measure and mitigate electromagnetic fields. The best way to determine your EMF exposure, and to monitor it over time, is to use an EMF meter (sold online at www .EMFSafetyStore.com).

- **Not getting enough sleep:** Your sleep can be affected by EMFs! Keep your bedroom as wireless-free as possible to prevent EMFs from disturbing your rest. I included an entire section on sleep later in this part (see page 245), so I'll just touch upon it here. Your body needs at least eight hours a night to rest and restore itself. Sure, a few restless nights are fine, but perpetually not getting enough sleep will take a toll on your physical and mental well-being.

Ask Carol

Can you suggest any supplements for aging well?

ANSWER:

First, I suggest getting your hair tested by your local holistic practitioner to see what kind of supplements you actually need. Just taking a general multivitamin may give you vitamins you don't need and may not give you enough of the vitamins your body lacks. Looking at your full health picture will help a nutritionist or doctor focus on which nutritional supplements you really need for optimal health.

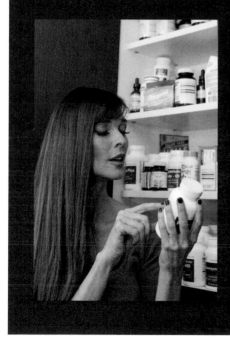

I take thirty different supplements three times a day, as well as herbs, kelp, chlorophyll, and digestive enzymes. Each person is different, so without testing it's hard to tell you exactly what supplements you would need. For me, anti-aging strategies are about giving the body everything it needs to rejuvenate and regenerate.

How to Age Gracefully

Now that we know the main factors that affect aging, what can we do to age gracefully? Unfortunately, we live in a youth-obsessed, very visually focused world. While many of us fear getting (and looking!) older, some women seem to get better and better with each passing year, like a fine wine! How is this? What do they have or do that's so different? I spoke to Susan Swimmer, an editor at *MORE* magazine, who shared some great tips with me on how to age gracefully:

IT'S ALL ABOUT CONFIDENCE

As you age, you should become more aware of who you are and what you love in life. You're free from the insecurities you had in your twenties, and the perfectionism of your thirties. It's time to feel confident in your own skin—trust me, it exudes from your pores!

LEARN TO LAUGH

Stop taking everything so seriously. Learn to laugh at yourself. "Laughter aids circulation, increases respiration, lowers blood pressure, stimulates digestion, and takes away stress and negativity," says Oz Garcia, PhD, a celebrity nutritionist and author of *Redesigning 50: The No-Plastic-Surgery Guide to 21st-Century Age Defiance*. A life without stress will last much longer.

ADJUST YOUR DIET AND EXERCISE

As you age, your metabolism slows down. A healthy diet and regular exercise can help with this, but you must be careful. If you gain three pounds a year beginning at age forty, by the time you're fifty-five, you'll be up forty-five pounds. Three pounds doesn't seem like a lot, but they add up over time, and it gets tougher and tougher to lose weight as you age. Maintenance is key!

AVOID YO-YO DIETING

Yo-yo dieting can actually be worse for you than not eating or over-eating. Think it's OK to skip meals some days and overeat on others? This eating pattern actually causes your body to get out of whack as your insulin and hormone levels constantly go up and down. Your body doesn't know how to handle these changes and is constantly in stress mode, which can lead to unwanted inflammation. It's best to stick to an overall healthy, real-food diet plan.

STAY INTERESTED AND ENGAGED

It's important to continue expanding your mind and cultivating your passions throughout life. Feeling burnt out? Find something new that interests you. Explore the world around you and constantly learn new things. We are lucky to live in a time where we can discover the world right at our fingertips. Go online and get inspired by a TED Talk, plan your next travel destination, learn French, or read the *New York Times*. The possibilities are endless!

Those are great tips from Susan! Educating myself about health living and now sharing everything I've learned with others has helped me keep my spark!

This sounds simple, but what happens when you are feeling down *all the time* and can't seem to pick yourself back up? Where did your energy go? And those moods! Enter perimenopause.

Perimenopause

Do you feel like you are already going through menopause and you're only in your thirties? Don't worry; you're not going crazy. Many women start to experience menopauselike symptoms in their early thirties and forties, including fatigue, unpredictable periods, hot flashes, roller-coaster emotions, and feeling bloated and even forgetful or fuzzy-minded. There's a lesser-known term for this stage *before* menopause: *perimenopause*.

Perimenopause can take a big toll on women's moods, health, and relationships. Suzanne Somers came on my show to discuss her book *I'm Too Young for This: The Natural Hormone Solution to Enjoy Perimenopause*. Suzanne hardly recognized herself at age thirty-five when she started to feel many of the symptoms I just described. They became unbearable and she went from doctor to doctor seeking help. Suzanne's health care providers didn't know what was going on and only offered her antidepressants, antianxiety and cholesterol-lowering medications, and diuretics. "Mood swings, PMS, plus annoying weight gain. I didn't know that these symptoms were simply a prelude to other changes I was about to experience," said Suzanne. "No one warned me I was about to lose 'me'!"

After years of no answers, Suzanne was finally able to find an endocrinologist who taught her that it was her hormones that were out of whack. Suzanne was estrogen dominant, and although most doctors told her not to take hormones, she realized what she was missing was progesterone. She needed more progesterone, the body's anticarcinogenic hormone, to balance out the estrogen.

Most women enter perimenopause between ages forty-five and fifty-five, but for some it starts as early as their midthirties. It can last anywhere from two years to ten. You're not officially in menopause until you've gone twelve months without a period, so many women find themselves in that middle ground.

Suzanne explained, "Perimenopause sneaks up on women because we are uneducated about our bodies. Our doctors are not up on hormonal changes in the female body. They think it's a temporary passage but nothing could be further from the truth. Once a woman or man begins declining in hormones it never stops, so replacement is in essence filling the tank for the rest of your life, as determined by lab work and your individual needs."

Hormones are crucial to life. The major hormones in the body are cortisol and other adrenal hormones, insulin, and thyroid hormones. The minor hormones are the sex hormones: estrogen, progesterone, and testosterone; they are usually the first to go, which causes an increase in the body's levels of the major hormones. The result is high levels of the stress hormone cortisol, which creates havoc in your body. The loss of minor hormones can also lead to high insulin levels, which will cause you to gain weight. Burnt-out adrenals create fatigue and many, many bodily problems. Suzanne found that the only way to deal with these shifting hormone levels was to take daily hormone supplements. This is a new treatment, so be sure to find a qualified doctor who can set you up with proper blood testing to determine your exact hormone needs. Suzanne suggests visiting www.ForeverHealth.com for more information.

Suzanne also suggested that eating properly helps immensely with perimenopause. You should know me by now! I'm all about the role that food and exercise play in maintaining a healthy body. Exercise also tells your cells that you are alive. All bodies need oxygenation.

Take a look at Suzanne's top fifteen power foods for perimenopause:

ALMONDS (RAW, UNSALTED)

Almonds are a great source of protein, fiber, and minerals, including:

Calcium and magnesium: Calcium keeps bones strong and promotes bone growth. Magnesium works in concert with calcium for bone growth and is a calming mineral needed by perimenopausal women. Magnesium nourishes the nervous system and helps prevent anxiety, nervousness, and irritability. It assists in relieving constipation.

Iron: This mineral is necessary for transporting the active and usable form of thyroid, T3, through the body.

Potassium: Circulatory deficits happen with age and declining hormones; potassium ameliorates this by helping to support blood vessel health and reduces the risk of high blood pressure. A potassium-rich diet will prevent leg cramps and other muscle spasms because of the role that potassium plays in muscle contraction and nerve impulses all over the body, including the heart.

Zinc: Research indicates that zinc helps balance the female hormones, helps prevent PMS, and helps prevent acne.

Almonds are also high in vitamin E and unsaturated fats, keeping arteries supple. With the decline of the minor hormones, the levels of major hormones, including cortisol, increase, which is one of the main causes of heart disease in women; almonds play a role in preventing atherosclerosis, the hardening of the arteries.

APPLES

All types of apples contain quercetin, a powerful antioxidant that prevents the oxidation of LDL cholesterol, which in turn lowers the risk of damage to your arteries. An apple's pectin is effective in lowering levels of LDL blood cholesterol.

BEANS

Beans are loaded with complex carbohydrates, as well as calcium, iron, folic acid, B vitamins, zinc, potassium, and magnesium. They contain large amounts of soluble and insoluble fiber, which helps reduce cholesterol and normalize blood sugar.

BEETS

Beets contain high levels of carotenoids and flavonoids, which are known to protect artery walls as well as reduce the risk of heart disease and stroke. In addition, they contain iron and calcium, which boosts bone health and reduces the risk of osteoporosis.

BLUEBERRIES

Berries are a great source of the antioxidants that keep your brain and heart healthy.

BROCCOLI

This vegetable contains two powerful anticancer substances: sulforaphane and indole-3-carbinol. Sulforaphane destroys ingested carcinogenic compounds and kills *H. pylori,* a bacterium that causes stomach ulcers and increases the risk of gastric cancers. (If you eat in restaurants and consume nonorganic chicken, it's likely at some point that you will pick up *H. pylori*.) Indole-3-carbinol metabolizes estrogen, which potentially protects against estrogen dominance and breast cancer. Broccoli also has a good amount of potassium and beta-carotene.

CABBAGE

High in fiber, vitamin A, and minerals, cabbage stimulates the immune system, kills bacteria and viruses, inhibits growth of cancerous cells, protects against tumors, helps control estrogen levels, promotes balance, improves blood flow, and boosts the sex drive. It speeds up the metabolism of estrogen toward a "good" metabolite and slows the production of a bad one, which reduces the risk of breast cancer; and it inhibits the growth of polyps in the colon. Cabbage also protects against stomach ulcers.

FLAXSEED

This power food increases the number of ovulatory cycles in perimenopausal women and increases testosterone at the time of ovulation. Regular consumption of flaxseed improves the progesterone-estrogen ratio in postovulatory women and helps with PMS. Flaxseed is also an excellent source of essential omega-3 fatty acids. Freshly ground flaxseed releases more nutrients than whole flaxseed, and the body is better able to digest ground flaxseed than the whole seed form.

GARLIC

This yummy bulb is an excellent cancer fighter, protecting against cancers of the breast, colon, skin, prostate, stomach, and esophagus. Garlic stimulates the immune system by encouraging the growth of natural killer cells that directly attack cancer cells. Also, it has the ability to kill many of the antibiotic-resistant strains of the hospital superbug MRSA.

NUTS AND SEEDS

Nuts and seeds provide excellent nutritional value. They are especially good sources of essential fatty acids, gamma tocopherol, vitamin E, protein, and minerals. They also provide valuable fiber components; important phytonutrients in nuts and seeds include protease inhibitors, ellagic acid, and other polyphenols.

OLIVE OIL

Regular consumption of this omega-3-rich oil helps protect against heart attacks, because of its unique polyphenol and monounsaturated fatty-acid content. Polyphenols in extra-virgin olive oil help keep cell membranes soft and pliable, allowing for oxygen and water, the elements of life, to flow through the membranes easily and thus add to cells' energy and vitality.

ORANGES

Oranges contain high quantities of hesperetin, which protects against inflammation. The fiber and pectin in this fruit can lower cholesterol. Oranges are a good source of potassium, which reduces blood pressure, as well as folic acid, which lowers levels of homocysteine (high levels of this substance are not good for the heart).

PINEAPPLE

This is one of the top fifty highest antioxidant content foods. Antioxidants have been found to help protect cells from the damage of free radicals, which can break down muscles, increase aging effects, and, as a result, lead to cancers and other chronic diseases.

SWEET POTATOES

This power food is full of protein, fiber, artery-protecting beta-carotene, blood pressure–controlling potassium, and antioxidants.

WILD SALMON

This fish is an excellent source of omega-3 fatty acids. Eating omega-3-rich salmon regularly may help protect against heart disease and breast and other cancers, as well as provide relief to sufferers of autoimmune diseases, such as rheumatoid arthritis and asthma. Its omega-3s are great for mood stability and also protect the brain, and are essential components of the membranes of every one of the sixty to ninety trillion cells in your body.

Fashion and Aging

As Susan Swimmer of *MORE* magazine explained earlier, confidence is a key component in feeling youthful and projecting that youthfulness to the world. As someone who's spent a lifetime working in the fashion industry, I've amassed quite a collection of fashion tips and advice, and I wanted to take some time to share that knowledge with women who are often overlooked and underserved in the fashion world.

There's no denying that our bodies change as we age. Like our hair and nails, our clothes also need to evolve as we get older. Style is about feeling confident in your own skin—but an amazing pair of jeans doesn't hurt either! I think women of all ages deserve to feel sexy and beautiful in the clothes they choose to wear! Remember, there is no age limit on good style.

Hopefully by the time you are in your thirties or forties you have defined your style and don't have to embrace every trend that comes

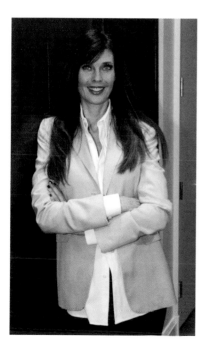

around. You know what works for your body type and have a few brands that you like. But you've probably fallen into a routine of wearing the same clothes you have worn for years. It's time to spice things up! You will feel better about yourself, and your spouse or partner is going to love this shake-up. Your body may not have the same shape or proportions it did ten years ago, and the styles of clothes that used to work for your body may no longer suit you—but remember that styles change and evolve with each new season. While you don't need to chase what twenty-year-olds may be wearing on the runway, you can, and should, have fun with style at every stage of your life.

The first step? Celebrity stylist and designer Phillip Bloch suggests—although every woman hates to hear this, myself included—cleaning out your closet! Phillip told me, "Twice a year, I suggest in the spring and fall, try on everything for that season and declutter your closet." I know it's hard to let go of all those shirts you will wear one day or the pants you will fit into if you just lose five pounds, but trust me, clothing selection will be much easier if everything in your closet fits you well . . . *right now.* It's better to have a few *wow* pieces than a full wardrobe of maybes. Donate those unworn clothes!

A big thing for me was buying only investment pieces. Stop spending twenty dollars on ten different shirts and instead buy one or two well-made shirts that fit you perfectly. When you are in your thirties or forties and beyond, it's time to wear better-quality clothes. You are at the point in life where buying poorly made pieces just doesn't make sense. A great-fitting blazer or blouse will add elegance to your look.

Carol's Tip

My favorite investment pieces are a special jacket (you will be wearing this every day in the winter!), a great-fitting blazer, stylish boots with only a small heel so you can walk in them, sunglasses, a nice scarf, and a great bag (that isn't too heavy itself—there's nothing worse than a bag that's heavy before you put anything in it!).

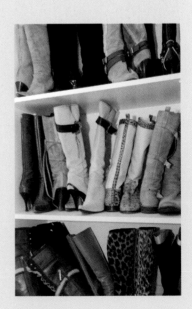

Ask Carol

Do you have any favorite fashion brands or wardrobe must-haves?

ANSWER:

I love the Italian brand Intimissimi's turtlenecks—they are light, stretchy, and soft, and they don't itch! I wear a lot of turtlenecks in the fall and winter. I find they look elegant under every jacket, and they're casual with jeans. They cover the neck and underarms. You can wear them loose fitting or tight depending on your body type. Check them out online at http://us.intimissimi.com.

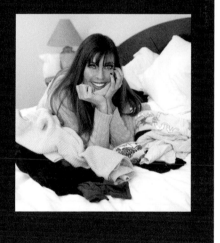

Want to know my secret for perfect legs? Berkshire Ultra Sheer toeless stockings.

Another secret? Tailor these clothes! Now that you've spent that money on those amazing pants—go to a tailor to make sure they fit you perfectly. According to Phillip Bloch, "Investing in tailoring your clothes makes all the difference in the world. All celebrities are doing this." Did you know Jennifer Aniston even tailors her T-shirts?

Phillip also recommends avoiding the sections of clothing stores targeted to older customers. Having more birthdays under your belt doesn't mean that you have to lose sight of your personal style and sense of fun when it comes to fashion. Limiting yourself to someone else's idea of age appropriateness will hinder your creativity. Instead, curate your own collection from all parts of the store. While you can embrace trends, go for a subtler version of what's hip—you'll look better in a more refined look, instead of an experimental or avant-garde runway look. Don't think this means you have to be boring, though.

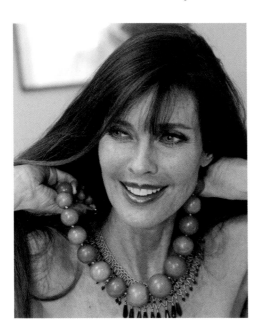

Another great fashion tip as you age is: wear those accessories! "A larger necklace can make you appear taller and leaner," Phillip added, because it directs attention up and away from your figure flaws. Accessories can help draw people's eyes to where you want them to look. I like to keep it simple with a great scarf or bag to complement my outfit. Scarves can do wonders and make any simple outfit look elegant and put together.

Carol's Tip

I find accessories are the most important part of getting dressed. You can take a moderately priced turtleneck and pair of jeans and build around them: add a great jacket, purse, shoes, coat, scarf, hat, or even a unique pair of gloves, and your outfit will instantly look classy and elegant.

Your Perfect Jeans

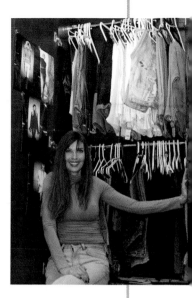

Everyone should have a pair of favorite jeans—you know the ones—the go-to pair that makes you feel sexy yet are super comfortable. These jeans should be currently in style and should flatter your best assets! The great news is that nowadays jeans companies are making jeans to accommodate every body type at every price point. So, as Phillip Bloch suggested, throw out those jeans from ten years ago that don't fit you right. It's silly to own five pairs of jeans that might fit one day. Instead, find one or two pairs that make you feel special and give you the wow factor right now.

I had Argy Koutsothanasis, a fashion director at *Fitness* magazine, share some tips on how to find the perfect pair of jeans.

Start out by knowing your body type. Are you a pear? Do you have a booty? Argy suggests you take notice of trends in fashion, but know what looks and makes you feel sexy and comfortable. She said, "We're all different—what's the point of wearing the latest trend if you have to keep pulling and tugging?"

Next, decide what color denim looks best on you. Argy recommended choosing darker denim as you age; it's slimming and offers a more sophisticated look. Next, check out the back and front pockets. Depending on the size of your derriere, pockets can do you wonders. Need a little oomph? Go with bigger pockets. Need to downsize? Go with smaller or no pockets. Also, be conscious of where they are placed—big, ill-placed pockets can accentuate your problem areas by making them look bigger or puffier. Trust me!

- **Don't buy jeans that are too tight.** This creates love handles and pushes your flesh to hang off your hip. Instead, if you are self-conscious about this area, opt for higher-waisted jeans to mask your problem areas.

- **Jeggings are a woman's best friend.** There's no point in being uncomfortable!

- **Wear thongs.** Panty lines can ruin your look.

- **Get your jeans hemmed.** Jeans are often too long for petite women. Instead of rolling them up, get them professionally hemmed. It's worth the investment.

- **Work it.** Only buy jeans you feel confident in! Confidence is the most important factor with any outfit.

Ask Carol

What is your favorite brand of jeans?

ANSWER:

My favorite jeans are Diesel or True Religion. I always wear straight-leg jeans because I like tucking them into my boots. I like jeans that come up just under my belly button, easily hiding any problem areas!

Are there any organic clothing brands that you would recommend?

ANSWER:

Nowadays in fashion, the words "eco-friendly," "organic," and "sustainable" get thrown around a lot. It can be hard to tell the difference between a brand that's actually helping to make the planet a better place—and one that's just riding the eco bandwagon.

Here are a few brands I've heard are great:

- LVR: Made here in the United States! (www.lvrfashion.com)

- My Tonic (http://mytonic.ca)

- Delikate Rayne (www.delikaterayne.com)

The Right Bra Can Change Your Life

One of the biggest clothing challenges for women can be finding the right bra. Many women wear the same kind and size for years, even when it no longer suits them or fits them correctly. Time to change it up!

Most women don't know what a bra should look like and how it should properly fit. In fact, according to style expert Brittney Levine, about 80 percent of women are wearing the wrong bra size! I'll be the first to admit that I was one of those women, before I became "bra-educated" myself. The bra is one of the most essential pieces in your wardrobe, so let's get it right!

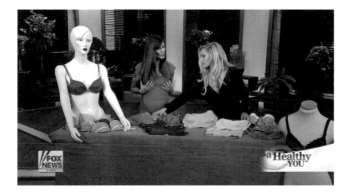

Brittney shared with us the biggest mistakes women make when buying bras and how to avoid them:

- **Choosing too large a band size.** Women often feel that they should buy a larger band size, but in actuality they should probably go down one size. If the band is too loose, the bra will not give you the correct support and lift. (Of course, if you find that the straps are digging into your shoulders, you definitely need to go up in band size.)

- **Choosing too small a cup size.** The most common problem Brittney sees is that women fear having a cup size high up in the alphabet. Women are known to choose bras that are three whole cup sizes too small for their bodies. A proper cup size ensures that all of the side breast tissue is scooped into the bra and helps women avoid spillage over the top. The A-to-D system is more than seventy years old and is not realistic by today's standards.

- **Ask the experts.** It can be embarrassing to get fitted by a complete stranger, but that's what the bra experts are there for! Most department or lingerie stores have a team of experts on hand just for this purpose. Ask for a fitting and let them help you pick styles that will work for your unique body. The best part: a fitting is usually free.

Women's bodies are constantly changing at different stages of their life—especially through pregnancy or during a significant weight gain or loss. It's a good idea to recycle your bras and get a new fitting every six months!

HOW TO CALCULATE BRA SIZE

1. **Determine your band size.** Using a measuring tape, measure the distance around your rib cage, just under your breasts. Round that measurement to the nearest whole number. You should measure yourself while braless and the tape should be snug and level. If the number is even, add 4 inches. If it's odd, add 5 inches.

   Your band size is the sum of the original measurement plus the add-on number. For example, if you measured

32 inches, your band size is 32 + 4 = 36. If you measured 33 inches, your band size is 33 + 5 = 38.

2. **Find your cup size**. Wrap the measuring tape somewhat loosely around the fullest part of your chest (at nipple level) to get your bust measurement. Round that measurement to the nearest whole number. Subtract your band size from your bust measurement and refer to the chart to find the corresponding cup letter. For example: 37 inches (bust) − 34 inches (band) = 3 inches. That's a 34C.

The difference (in inches)	0	1	2	3	4	5	6	7
Your cup size	AA	A	B	C	D	DD	DDD & F	G

BRA TIPS FOR EVERY BODY TYPE

- If you have narrow shoulders, try a cross-back or multiway style.
- If you have a broad back, you may prefer balcony shapes.
- If your breasts are wide-set, try a low-cut balcony shape.
- If your breasts are close-set, try a plunge or push-up shape.
- If one breast is larger than the other, try a T-shirt bra with a pad in the cup of your smaller breast. Always fit a bra to your fuller breast.

- If your breasts have lost tone, look for balcony styles with slight padding that will give you shape and support.

It's important to wear the right undergarments as a foundation for your look. There's nothing worse than having great clothes on but having to adjust your bra strap all day! Invest in the right-size bra—it makes all the difference.

Carol's Tip

Wear nonunderwire bras! According to Tammy Kohlschmidt, RDH, CCT, CBP, studies have shown that wearing an underwire bra raises the temperature of your breasts and restricts oxygen and nutrient flow to the breast tissues. Wearing an underwire bra also restricts the flow of toxin-removing lymphatic drainage. Aluminum from antiperspirants, for example, is one potentially dangerous source of toxins that can accumulate if your lymph drainage is impaired. The pressure that bras put on this system can cause a congestion of toxins, which leads to fluid buildup, swelling, tenderness, and cyst formation.

Osteoporosis

Now that you're feeling good about your outer appearance, let's get back to your inner! It's important to pay attention to your bone health as you age. As you get older, your bones tend to shrink in size and density. This weakens them and makes them more susceptible to fracture. Remember how Grandma used to be taller than you and is now under your chin?

Osteoporosis is a condition in which the bones become fragile because of bone density loss. The symptoms are often back pain, stooped posture, loss of height, and easily fractured bones. Stress, poor nutrition, and highly acidic blood all deplete calcium stores; as a result, the body leaches calcium from the bones.

I had Mira Calton, nutritionist and coauthor of *Naked Calories*, on *A Healthy You & Carol Alt* to discuss bone health with me. Mira suffered from osteoporosis, but with the help of her husband, Dr. Jayson Calton, a specialist in the field, she was able to reverse it. Here's how.

Many people believe that only older people get osteoporosis. Mira was under the same illusion, until at age thirty she was told she had the bones of an eighty-year-old. It was a quick decline for her. One day she was twenty-nine, living in New York City where she was the lead publicist of her own public relations firm, and the next day she was battling for her health. At first she started to feel a throbbing around her hips and lower back. "I just blamed it on my stilettos and too many late nights out with clients," she explained. The pain finally got so bad that Mira would spend days lying on her sofa with her computer on her chest, just trying to work. After turning thirty she went to a doctor who told her she had advanced osteoporosis, that it would never get better, and that "my family would have to take care of me."

Mira knew this wasn't the life she wanted for herself. She was a young, vibrant professional, and she refused to accept the fate her doctor had described to her. So she went to visit another doctor, Jayson Calton, now her husband, to see how her diet was affecting her bones. Together, they developed a program called micronutrient therapy, which pinpoints vitamin and mineral deficiencies, and explores how they can affect your health.

Mira learned that the body requires certain essential micronutrients to be healthy, so she and Jayson created a simple three-step plan to address her osteoporosis. She mapped out the plan for me:

STEP ONE:
SWITCH TO MICRONUTRIENT-RICH FOOD

Before I changed my diet I was under the impression that I was eating healthy food. Wow, did I have a lot to learn! Little did I know that my diet of fat-free muffins for breakfast, spinach salads for lunch, and low-fat, steamed Chinese food for dinner was literally robbing me of my bone health. Now, Jayson and I teach people how to identify micronutrient-rich food that will boost their metabolisms and fill their bodies with the essential micronutrients they need to protect their health and enable them to function at peak performance levels at work and play.

High-quality foods supply greater amounts of these important vitamins and minerals. Simply switching to micronutrient-rich foods from poor, micronutrient-depleted foods with dangerous additives can assure you greater micronutrient intake. For example, pasture-raised hens, which are allowed free access to grass and insects, produce eggs that contain up to ten times more omega-3s, and three to six times more vitamin D than eggs from factory-farmed hens raised in confinement. This simple food swap packs a ton more micronutrients in every bite.

STEP TWO:
DRIVE DOWN DEPLETION

It is also imperative to identify something we call everyday micro-nutrient depleters (EMDs)—dietary and lifestyle habits that may be directly robbing you of micronutrients and the optimal health you deserve. I had to learn to avoid numerous EMDs hiding in foods—such as phosphoric acid (often found in soda), sugar (hiding everywhere these days), and phytic and oxalic acids found in grains, beans, and some greens such as spinach—in order to make sure they were not depleting my bones of calcium, magnesium, and vitamin D. Additionally, I changed my high-intensity cardiovascular workouts to weight-bearing workouts to avoid excess mineral loss through sweat and to stimulate bone growth. I had to identify the over-the-counter or pre-scription medications I was taking that might affect my micronutrient sufficiency levels. I also had to adjust my stress levels, moderate my love of red wine, and even look more closely at the household toxins that existed in my home. It was eye opening and really made me aware of how many things we all encounter every day that can deplete us of the micronutrients we need to maintain our health.

STEP THREE:
UTILIZE SMART SUPPLEMENTATION

The body simply cannot function without proper micronutrient nour-ishment, but in our modern world of vitamin- and -mineral-depleted soil, factory farming, and global food manufacturing, our food is simply not supplying us with adequate amounts of these essential micronutrients. It is important to supplement smartly by utilizing a well-formulated custom supplementation program that the body can really absorb. It should contain the highest-quality vitamins and minerals, delivered in such a way as to avoid the innate competitions between nutrients that too often eliminate the positive benefits that they promise to deliver. To help people make sense of supplement labels and find products that really work, Jayson and I created a free educational video series, which can be viewed at www.ABCsofSupplementation.com.

Mira is now happy and healthy, with strong bones, and inspiring others to follow what she did so they can feel the same! The Caltons have written a new book, *The Micronutrient Miracle,* which explains their signature twenty-eight-day micronutrient therapy program for disease prevention, as well as eight other more personalized, condition-specific protocols for osteoporosis, fat loss, cardiovascular health, blood sugar regulation, hormone regulation, digestive health, autoimmune conditions, and an advanced ketogenic protocol. Check out the book for more information on this important topic!

Your Sex Life After Menopause

Menopause is often characterized by hot flashes and mood swings. But these are not the only changes a woman goes through during and after this life stage. It can be taboo to talk about it, but many women also suffer from a loss of interest in sex or experience pain during sex after menopause. While it may seem embarrassing to bring it up at the doctor's office or with your partner, you're not alone in this! Menopause-related sexual issues are far more common than you'd imagine. You should never be afraid to ask for help—there are solutions available that could make a positive difference in your life.

The loss of estrogen and testosterone during menopause can lead to changes in a woman's body and sex drive. Many menopausal and postmenopausal women notice that they're not as easily aroused, and they may be less interested in sex. Also, lower levels of estrogen often cause a drop in blood supply to the vagina. That affects vaginal lubrication, causing the vagina to be too dry for comfortable sex—but there's help for that.

While it's a sensitive topic for some, Oscar-nominated actress Virginia Madsen spoke to me about this problem, which is called dyspareunia, and is caused by an atrophied uterine wall. Virginia, who is perimenopausal, said her mother and sister experienced menopause very differently from each other. She wanted to see what was in store for her, but found a limited amount of information on the subject available to her. As noted earlier, perimenopause refers to the years leading up to menopause, and although Virginia didn't experience hot flashes per se, she often felt herself heating up and becoming warm. She also found that she was forgetful and had trouble concentrating.

Virginia's advice: Although sexual problems can be hard to discuss, it's important to talk to your doctor if you are experiencing any side effects of menopause. To help with the pain of dyspareunia, head right to your kitchen and grab some coconut oil. (You can use this stuff for everything!) There are also great natural lubricants on the market, such as FORIA or Sylk. You know me, I recommend always going with the natural option! Sex should always be enjoyable and doesn't need to be something you stop doing as you age and your body changes. The *Journal of the American Geriatrics Society* recently revealed a healthy sex life could be the secret to living a long, happy life. Don't miss out!

Who Needs Sleep? You Do!

Another important secret to aging well is getting enough sleep every night. Studies associate sleep deprivation with weight gain, diabetes, cardiovascular ailments, and even increased cancer risk.

How much sleep our bodies need varies with age, but health experts suggest 7.5 to 8 hours per night, with children and teenagers sometimes needing more. Insufficient quality ZZZs can result in:

- **Obesity:** Lack of sleep makes us more prone to making bad food choices. When you're tired, you tend to reach for anything to satisfy your hunger, instead of preparing healthy meals and snacks. Not to mention you won't feel much like exercising.

  More than that, sleep is connected to hormones that regulate appetite, stress, and energy. One of these, leptin, suppresses appetite and moderates energy balance, but it's decreased with sleep deprivation.

- **Immune function:** Sleep deprivation kills off immune cells, putting you at greater risk of inflammation, which leads to disease (like some cancers) and aging.

So now that you know why it's important to get a full night's rest, here's what you can do to get more satisfying slumber:

- **Establish a pre-bedtime ritual.** Take a warm bubble bath, meditate, or read. These activities allow you to slow down and tell your body it's almost time to sleep.

- **Stay away from all electronics an hour before bedtime.** The light exposure before sleep can disrupt body rhythms and suppress the release of the hormone melatonin.

- **Check your mattress and box spring.** Is it comfortable and in good shape, or worn out? If it's looking saggy and unsupportive, consider a new set. Never ignore the box spring; that's the foundation of your sleep station. I prefer natural fiber mattresses. Who wants to sleep on chemicals? I worry about the harmful effects of breathing them in all night.

- **Think about when you eat.** Give yourself a chance to digest before bedtime by eating at least three hours before. If you feel full when you go to bed, try digestive enzymes to help soothe your stomach.

Carol's Tip

I use a little bit of Saint John's-wort and melatonin when I have trouble sleeping. Another solution that works for me is a little bit of lavender mixed with olive oil rubbed under my nose. Not only does it moisturize, but it can relax you with every breath!

Sleep troubles might also be caused by low magnesium levels. Before you go to bed, try taking some magnesium. I recommend Natural Calm from Natural Vitality.

Also, try sleeping with a pillow between your legs. This helps with proper spinal alignment.

I hope I've helped you realize that aging is actually a great thing. If you eat properly, exercise, and take care of yourself, you will not only reap the benefits of a healthy lifestyle, but you'll also become more self-aware and confident as you get older. When we are younger we tend to focus on ego-driven superficial pursuits—our appearance, making lots of money, accumulating material things, and acting a certain way toward others. But as you get older you learn what's truly important and valuable in life—your relationships, family, meaningful work, interesting and fulfilling experiences, continued growth and learning, and joy in simple things.

Engage with the world as you embrace each year that passes, and always focus on what's truly important in your life—health, happiness, and years of continued growth, laughter, and fun!

Final Thoughts

*I*t seems to me that most people I meet would love to be healthy, on some level. Sure, there are some people who just enjoy indulging in vices every day, and there are those who have uncontrollable self-destructive streaks, but for the vast majority of us, optimal health is a goal we strive to attain.

If you're not at the place you'd like to be when it comes to your diet or fitness routines, what's holding you back? Even though we all know we should be making healthy decisions, sometimes the excuses just take over and block out our thought processes. Self-talk like "I can't resist this one dessert" and "I'll quit smoking next week" and "I'll join a gym in the new year" becomes a real-life roadblock that gets in the way of our best intentions.

If there is one takeaway from this book, let it be this: do not allow the excuses—the daily time crunch or the family obligations or the pile of work projects—to prevent you from making smart, positive decisions. Start now. Go look at yourself in the mirror and tell yourself this very minute that you are going to eat better and exercise and head down the path of looking and feeling the best you possibly can. If you are disciplined, this does not have to be a 100 percent, all-or-nothing choice. You can still splurge on unhealthy, tasty treats on occasion; you can take a day off from exercise as needed. But I promise those small breaks and lapses will start to become fewer and fewer as you begin to notice how you feel on the days when you are focusing on your health. Once you start to see positive changes in the way you look and feel inside and out, you won't want to stop. So take a leap of faith and set out on the road to a healthy you! You won't regret it.

Acknowledgments

I'd like to thank the many important people who have helped me along on my own personal journey to better health!

To Roger Ailes, without your incredible insight and unwavering confidence in me, there would be no *A Healthy You & Carol Alt* or the incredible opportunity to turn the show into this book!

To Laura Dail, my patient and persistent literary agent! You've kept everything moving and never lost faith—ever! Six books and counting!

To my manager, Scott Hart, who has always been there for me, but especially on this book. Thanks for always being there to listen. A book, any book, is never easy! Whether it's the first or the sixth, it's equally tough.

To Jocelyn Steiber, who took on the immense task of delivering this book under great pressure. You did unbelievably!!! I couldn't have asked for more from you.

To my mom, Muriel Alt, and my sisters, Karen Roos and Christine Gratowski, and my boyfriend, Alexei Yashin, for supporting me always.

To Bill Shine, Suzanne Scott, and John Finley, for working with me on the show and turning the other cheek when I really wanted to do something crazy, different, and alternative. In other words: nuts!

To Jessica Dymczyk, Loren Petterson, Joan McNaughton, Tyla Tyus, and Jennings Grant, for lifting me up every day so I look better, sound better, and present better—I'm better because of you all.

To my wonderful photographers, Antoine Verglas, Sunny Bak, and Jimmy Bruch, thank you! And to HarperCollins, for seeing the value of the collected wisdom from *A Healthy You & Carol Alt*: especially Brittany Hamblin, Lynn Grady, Heidi Richter, and Kendra Newton. Thank you all for your help and patience. I hope this book and I live up to your expectations.

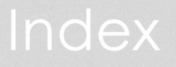

Index

Photography Credits